the alli diet

Your essential guide to success with alli

HARPER

HARPER

an imprint of HarperCollins*Publishers*
77–85 Fulham Palace Road,
Hammersmith, London W6 8JB

www.harpercollins.co.uk

First published by HarperCollins*Publishers* 2009
This edition 2011

10 9 8 7 6 5 4 3 2 1

A catalogue record of this book is
available from the British Library

ISBN 978-0-00-729372-8

Printed and bound in Great Britain by
Clays Ltd, St Ives plc

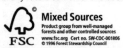

Mixed Sources
Product group from well-managed
forests and other controlled sources
www.fsc.org Cert no. SW-COC-001806
© 1996 Forest Stewardship Council

the alli diet

Contents

Chapter 1   What is **alli**?   1

Chapter 2   Your Diet Essentials   17

Chapter 3   The Menu Plans   30

Chapter 4   Recipes   60

Breakfasts and Brunches   65
Soups   77
Sandwiches and Light Lunches   89
Main Course Salads   105
Poultry   117
Meat   139
Fish and Seafood   173
Vegetarian   197
Sides   209
Pasta   225
Sauces, Dressings and Dips   237
Desserts   253
Bites   275
Recipes by kcal per portion   286
Recipes by fat per portion   289

Chapter 5	Eating Out	293
Chapter 6	Going Shopping	310
Chapter 7	Exercise	320
Chapter 8	Keep Going!	331
Chapter 9	Portion Guide and Calorie-counter	335

Chapter 1

What is **alli**?

Successful Weight-loss Starts Here

Losing weight will not only help you to feel better in yourself, it will also reduce your health risks. Sounds obvious, doesn't it?

However, it's no secret that losing weight can be really hard work. In spite of knowledge and determination, it can be a real struggle to lose weight and keep it off.

That's why **alli** is an exciting development for adults who are overweight, with a BMI of 28 or above, and who want to make positive changes to their weight. It isn't a miracle pill or a crash diet; it's the first pharmacy-only weight-loss aid to be licensed for use throughout Europe. Also available is the **alli** support programme to guide you towards your weight-loss goal.

Adding **alli** to a reduced calorie, lower-fat diet is clinically proven to help you lose 50% more weight. So for every 2 lb (1 kg) you lose from dieting, **alli** can help you lose an extra 1 lb (0.5 kg).

The **alli** programme is a sensible approach to losing weight which helps you commit to lasting, positive changes to your eating and lifestyle habits.

How Is **alli** Different?

alli is a clinically proven weight-loss aid that should be combined with a reduced-calorie, lower-fat diet. You should also try to introduce more activity into your daily life. The **alli** programme can help you break your old habits and follow a healthier lifestyle.

alli works by attaching itself to some of the enzymes that break down fat. This stops about a quarter of the fat you eat from being digested and absorbed, so the unabsorbed fat passes naturally out of the body.

When you take **alli**, you have the reassurance that it is the first pharmacy-only weight-loss aid licensed throughout Europe.

With **alli**, you also have the reassurance of knowing that it's been extensively studied in clinical trials.

Visit www.**alli**.co.uk for more information. Remember to read the label and the information leaflet in the **alli** pack before you start.

What Is **alli**?

alli is a capsule taken with a reduced-calorie, lower-fat diet.

alli is not a quick fix or a miracle pill. As we all know, quick fixes never work.

The **alli** programme requires you to make simple but significant changes to your eating habits. It also recommends that you combine these changes with a more active lifestyle.

It shows you how to make positive, long-term changes in your life and provides you with essential tools and techniques so you can keep the weight off.

How Does **alli** Work?

- In order to digest the food you eat, your body releases natural enzymes.
- There are different enzymes to break down proteins, carbohydrates and fats.
- **alli** contains orlistat which only works on the enzymes that break down fat, so proteins and carbohydrates aren't affected and you can absorb all of these nutrients.
- As **alli** can lower the levels of some vitamins absorbed by your body, you should take a multivitamin containing vitamins A, D, E and K every

day at bedtime (when you will not be taking **alli**) to help ensure the vitamins are absorbed.

- **alli** stops the enzymes digesting about a quarter of the fat you eat. As the undigested fat can't be absorbed, it passes naturally out of the body.
- Fat is the most calorie-dense food, so preventing the absorption of some of it with **alli** and eating reduced-calorie, lower-fat meals helps you lose weight.

Diet-related Treatment Effects

Since **alli** works on the enzymes in your body to prevent some of the fat you eat from being absorbed, if you eat too much fat at any one time, you may notice some bowel changes. These are known as diet-related treatment effects and can include any of the following:

- fatty or oily stools
- loose, soft stools
- sudden bowel motions
- wind (flatulence) with or without oily spotting.

Controlling the fat content of your meals will help you avoid these effects.

It's really a very simple equation: as **alli** prevents the absorption of about a quarter of the fat you eat, if you eat a chicken meal containing 15g of fat, 4g of undigested fat passes out of your body. In the same way, if you eat a hamburger meal containing 80g of fat, you will pass 20g of undigested fat.

Therefore, any diet-related treatment effects can be minimized by keeping within the recommended amounts of fat per meal and snack.

Your Signal

The surplus fat that passes naturally out of your body is simply undigested fat. If you experience any of the diet-related treatment effects, this is a signal that you have eaten a meal or snack that may have contained more fat than the recommended fat target. Please refer to the tables further on in this book for more information on recommended fat targets.

Tips for Avoiding Diet-related Treatment Effects

Managing diet-related treatment effects is an important part of making **alli** work for you. Here are some tips to help you stay in control.

- Start your lower-fat diet a few days, or even a week, before you begin taking the capsules.
- Find out more about how much fat your favourite foods typically contain and the size of your portions (check the labels). By getting used to more appropriate portion sizes, you'll be less likely to accidentally go over your fat target.
- Distribute your fat allowance evenly across your meals for the day. Don't 'save' fat grams from lunch and 'spend' them at dinner – each meal and snack must be within your fat target.
- Be patient. It may take a little time to familiarize yourself with your fat and calorie targets. Most users who experience diet-related treatment effects at the start learn how to reduce them.
- Keeping a food diary is an invaluable tool for helping you to recognize which foods can lead to diet-related treatment effects. Jot down helpful notes and favourite recipes – you'll soon get into the swing of things.

Is **alli** Right For Me?

alli is for people who are ready and willing to make the necessary adjustments to their lifestyle. If you are an overweight adult aged 18 or over with a Body Mass Index (BMI) of 28 or over, **alli** can help you to lose weight. Visit www.**alli**.co.uk to work out your BMI.

    alli is an effective weight loss aid, but it's not suitable for everyone. Talk to your pharmacist to determine whether **alli** is right for you. Make sure you also read the information contained in the **alli** pack before you start taking **alli**.

    alli is already helping thousands of people lose weight and make positive changes to their lifestyle. You too could enjoy success with **alli** if you're willing to make some simple, long-lasting changes to your eating habits. Your commitment is the key to your success.

Losing weight doesn't happen overnight, so **alli** and the **alli** programme encourages gradual, steady weight loss of 1–2 lb (0.5–1 kg) a week. The **alli** programme can inspire and teach you to adopt healthier eating habits. Step by step you can do it with **alli**.

Losing even a modest amount of weight can significantly reduce the risk of developing several serious health problems, such as diabetes and heart disease. If you are concerned about the risks associated with being over-weight, see your doctor for a check-up.

How to Take **alli**

Take one capsule, three times a day at mealtimes – this usually means one at breakfast, lunch and dinner. (Remember to make these meals well balanced, reduced calorie and lower-fat.)

Take **alli** just before, during or up to one hour after meals. Swallow the capsule whole with water.

If you miss a meal, or your meal doesn't contain fat, don't take a capsule – **alli** doesn't work unless there's some fat in the meal.

Do not take more than 3 capsules a day.

Remember also to take a multivitamin tablet at bedtime (containing vitamins A, D, E and K). As **alli** removes some of the fat you eat from your body, some fat-soluble vitamins are removed with it. Taking a daily multivitamin ensures that you have an adequate supply of these vital nutrients.

Adjusting to Your New Lifestyle

There are a few simple but fundamental changes you will need to make in your life to succeed with the **alli** programme.

Here's what you need to be willing to do to join the thousands who are succeeding with **alli**:

- adopt a reduced-calorie, lower-fat diet
- plan your meals
- manage your cravings and setbacks
- take guidance from the **alli** programme.

Achieving your goal with **alli** isn't complicated; it just takes a little practice to get into the new habits. As well as sticking to a reduced-calorie, lower-fat diet, becoming more physically active is part and parcel of becoming healthier. Like most things in life, once you're used to them, they simply become part of your daily routine.

Commit to a Reduced-calorie, Lower-fat Diet

Why Reduce Calories?

Calories are a measurement of the energy your body needs to function. When you eat more calories than your body needs, it stores the excess energy as fat.

Your calorie target is the maximum number of calories you should eat per day. This target varies, according to your weight, gender and activity levels. You can use the chart (below) to set your daily calorie targets.

Before you can set your calorie targets you'll need to know your activity level. The more active you are, the higher your calorie limit. Choose which activity level most closely fits your daily routine. If you're unsure which is your level, choose 'low'.

- Low activity = you do little or no walking, stair-climbing, gardening or other physical activity on a daily basis
- Moderate activity = you burn around 150 calories a day in physical activity, for example, walking 2 miles (3 kilometres), gardening for 30–45 minutes, or running 1.25 miles (2 kilometres) in 15 minutes.

Calories for Women

Low Activity	Below 68.1kg	Below 10st 10lb	1200 calories
	68.1kg to 74.7kg	10st 10lb to 11st 11lb	1400 calories
	74.8kg to 83.9kg	11st 12lb to 13st 2lb	1600 calories
	84.0kg and over	13st 3lb and over	1800 calories
Moderate Activity	Below 61.2kg	Below 9st 9lb	1400 calories
	61.3kg to 65.7kg	9st 9lb t0 10st 4lbs	1600 calories
	65.8kg and over	10st 5lb and over	1800 calories

Calories for Men

Low Activity	Below 65.7kg	Below 10st 4lb	1400 calories
	65.8kg to 70.2kg	10st 5lb to 11st	1600 calories
	70.3kg and over	11st 1lb and over	1800 calories
Moderate Activity	59.0kg and over	9st 4lb and over	1800 calories

Lower Fat Is Key

You may be surprised to know that **alli** doesn't require you to eliminate fat completely from your diet. Eating the right amount of fat helps the body absorb vitamins and perform other essential functions.

Your fat target is the maximum amount of fat each meal and snack should contain for you as an individual while on the **alli** programme. This is based on your daily calorie intake. When you follow the **alli** programme, you'll be focusing on the **total** amount of fat, not whether it's unsaturated or saturated.

Use the chart below to set your fat target for each meal and snack.

	1200kcal		1400kcal		1600kcal		1800kcal	
	kcal	fat g	Kcal	fat g	kcal	fat g	kcal	fat g
Breakfast	300	<12	350	<15	400	<17	450	<19
Lunch	350	<12	400	<15	500	<17	550	<19
Dinner	400	<12	500	<15	550	<17	650	<19
Snack	150	<3	150	<3	150	<3	150	<3
Total	1200	39	1400	48	1600	54	1800	60

Reducing fat not only helps you to lose weight, it is also the way that you will be able to manage any diet-related treatment effects such as fatty or oily stools, sudden bowel motions and wind (flatulence). These effects are caused by the way the **alli** capsules work on the food you eat: because **alli** prevents the absorption of some of the fat in the food you eat, this unabsorbed fat passes naturally out of the body. Be reassured that most new **alli** users who experience these effects learn how to manage them by staying within their recommended fat targets.

Tastier, Healthier Food

alli is dedicated to helping you eat a tasty, nutritious and varied diet. Although it's important to limit the foods that are high in fat and calories, there are lots of other delicious choices open to you.

Lower-fat doesn't have to mean lower-taste; we have lots of easy, satisfying recipes and meal ideas to prove it. The advice in this book should enable you to eat satisfying, balanced meals without feeling bored or deprived.

Enjoy trying new things and varying your meals with **alli**.

Eating Together

With the **alli** programme you will be able to eat such a variety of delicious food that your whole family can enjoy the same meals as you. Some of the recipes are written for two, some for more, and many are adaptations of family favourites.

At the Table

Putting the right amount of the right foods on your plate is a simple but important part of achieving success.

Try downsizing your plate to downsize your portions. If you use a plate that's 20cm (8 inches) across, it'll look fuller so you won't feel you're missing out.

When you're sure of your portion sizes at home, you'll then find it easier to judge how much you should eat when you dine out (restaurants usually serve bigger portions than you need).

Planning Your Meals

Ideally, you will plan your meals while you're on the **alli** programme so you can stay within your recommended fat target per meal. Knowing what you're going to eat a few days in advance puts you in control and raises your chances of success. Planning ahead helps you avoid making last-minute choices which are too high in fat and calories. It also enables you to experiment with new recipes.

In reality, you probably won't be able to plan every meal. However, as you learn more about the programme you should be able to assess what will and won't work within the programme for you. This book will help.

Shopping

Try not to go shopping when you're hungry. You could be tempted by fatty convenience foods and may start snacking on your way home.

Also, if you don't already make shopping lists, start now and try to stick to them.

There are lots more tips on better (and smarter) shopping later in the book.

Move Your Body and Shift the Weight

The **alli** programme recommends you increase your physical activity levels to help you lose more weight.

When you consume fewer calories your body has to use its fat stores for energy and, as it does that, you lose pounds. When you exercise, you encourage your body to burn fat stores more often and, as a result, help increase your weight loss. Upping your activity levels should help you lose more weight.

Incorporating more physical activity into your everyday life is easier than you think. There are lots of fun and easy ways to exercise.

Exercising isn't just good for your body, it's a well-known fact that it's good for your mood and relieves stress, too. It's not just about joining a gym; there are lots of other ways to get moving and burn calories.

Whatever shape you're in and however busy you are, it's still possible to be active every day. Start gently and increase slowly. Begin with 10 minutes' extra walking a day. If you're already active, then build up the time or add in something else as well.

Remember to check with your doctor before you start any new exercise programme.

There's a chapter on exercising as part of the **alli** programme later in the book, but here are some tips to get you thinking about how to include more activity in your daily life:

- Write your goals down somewhere you will see them every day.
- Break your goal into long-term and short-terms goals that are achievable.
- Involve family and friends in your weight-loss plan.
- Take the stairs more often at home – make extra trips and burn extra calories.
- Don't sit down when you make a phone call – walk about the house while you talk.
- Cleaning is good: hoovering, mopping and dusting are all excellent activities for burning fat.
- Take a seat on an exercise ball. It will help you sit up straight and work your abdominal muscles.
- Get off the bus one stop early. When you feel ready you can try two stops earlier!
- Cycle rather than driving whenever you can.
- Walk up escalators.
- If you take the lift, get out a floor early or take the stairs from ground level.
- Park further from the shops and walk the rest of the way there. Supermarket car parks can be huge, so get into the habit of parking as far away from the shop entrance as possible.
- Walk the dog! A brisk daily walk will help burn off any extra calories consumed.
- Get gardening – a great way to burn some extra calories.

Managing Cravings …

Cravings can be the downfall of many dieters.

It's important to learn, therefore, to recognize whether your body is hungry or if you're experiencing a craving for something. Hunger is an empty feeling in your stomach – a signal that you haven't eaten anything for several hours. A craving doesn't mean that your body is hungry; it usually happens when you feel like eating a certain type of food. It can be triggered by stimuli outside the body, such as stress, changes in emotions and seeing or smelling something appetizing.

It would be unrealistic to tell you that you won't experience cravings, but it is possible to control them and limit the damage they can cause.

Tips for Beating Cravings

- Drink a glass or two of water – sometimes your body is thirsty and not hungry at all.
- If you feel like chocolate, whisk up a cup of reduced-calorie hot chocolate with water or skimmed milk and a shake of cinnamon on top.
- If you're at home, do something to take your mind off the craving – walking away from the fridge and out of the kitchen is a good start! You could try phoning a friend, doing 10 star jumps or taking up knitting to distract yourself.

… and Setbacks

Blips. Bumps in the road. Snack-attacks. Whatever you call them, they happen to everyone. The essential factor is how you handle the setback.

If you eat the wrong foods and/or too much of them, don't be too hard on yourself because that can make things worse. Instead, accept that it's happened and decide why, so you can aim to avoid the same mistake again.

- After a setback, make your next meal really tasty and within the accepted fat and calorie limits.
- Then start planning an occasion or night out and make a shopping list of the new, smaller clothes you'd like to buy for it to spur yourself on.

Take Support from the **alli** Programme

When you commit to the **alli** programme, it's committed to you. It's here to help you adopt a healthy lifestyle so you can reach your goals.

Visit www.**alli**.co.uk for online support, useful tools, tips and more recipes to help you stay motivated and on track.

Are You Ready?

Before you start, here are some final things to remember:

- Don't rush: **alli** provides you with a gradual and steady approach to weight loss. You can use **alli** for up to six months.
- Smaller portions = a bigger reward. If you commit to a healthy lifestyle, following a reduced calorie, lower-fat diet, **alli** can reward your hard work with 50% more weight loss. So, for every 2 lb you lose by your own efforts, **alli** can help you lose 1 lb more.
- Lower-fat is the way forward: limiting the amount of fat you eat at each meal is very important when you're taking **alli** capsules. If you don't stick to it, you increase your chances of experiencing diet-related treatment effects.
- Get more physically active: Exercise helps to burn calories, so when you're taking **alli**, you can help yourself by taking more exercise.
- Remember to read the label and information leaflet that comes with the **alli** pack before you start.

Your Reward

Successful weight loss may seem like a big challenge, but **alli** can be a big help. Importantly, the **alli** programme provides you with useful tools to help you sustain your weight loss and commit to lasting, positive changes to your eating and lifestyle habits.

This is the first step on your journey to a healthier lifestyle. Good luck!

Fiona Wilcock MSc BA PGCE RPHNutr

Chapters 2, 3, 4, 5, 6, 8 and 9 have been written by Fiona Wilcock, an independent nutrition consultant with extensive experience in the field of food and nutrition. She has a degree in Home Economics and five years' teaching experience, first in the UK then at Egerton University in Kenya. After returning to the UK from Kenya, Fiona completed an MSc in Nutrition at King's College London before working for the British Nutrition Foundation.

Now freelance, Fiona provides nutrition training and technical support to a number of organizations, in both the public and private sector. She has worked with Marks & Spencer over many years, writing menu plans for their food ranges and providing technical advice and training.

Fiona has written widely on diet and health for a range of organizations, including the Food and Health Alliance, Scotland, and the Health Education Board for Scotland, as well as developing recipes and nutrition information for BabyCentre and Healthy Living websites. She is the author of *The Complete Pregnancy Cookbook*, winner of the Gourmand Cookbook Award for the Best Health and Nutrition Book in the UK in 2002, which has been printed in ten languages and was revised and reprinted in 2008. As the nutrition expert for *Mother & Baby* magazine she provided advice on diet in pregnancy and early years.

Chapter 7 has been written by Ann-See Yeoh of FitPro, which is the largest and most respected association for fitness industry professionals in the world, with over 75,000 members. Ann-See Yeoh, MMedSci, is FitPro's Curriculum Manager. She holds a masters degree in Sport & Exercise Science and has lectured on undergraduate and postgraduate Sports Science courses for 8 years. In this role she established key links between the university and the fitness industry, as well as a major local obesity clinic. Prior to working for FitPro, Ann-See has been instrumental in developing and tutoring a wide range of courses within the fitness industry She is an international presenter and trainer.

Acknowledgements

Fiona Wilcock would particularly like to acknowledge the help of the following people in providing nutrition information for the book:

Charlotte Parker, company nutritionist at Sainsbury's
Claire Hughes, company nutritionist at Marks & Spencer
Moira Howie, company nutritionist at Waitrose
Laura Street, nutritionist at Tesco
Victoria Pennington, company nutritionist at Boots

Thanks too to Tinuviel software, whose program WISP was used to do all the recipe and menu-plan analysis.

More importantly, thanks are also due to my family for being willing guinea pigs as the recipes were tested, and for patience as I completed the book.

Chapter 2

Your Diet Essentials

Well done for taking the first steps to a healthier, trimmer you. The information in this chapter will help you learn how to eat a healthier diet, both while you are trying to lose weight and in the longer term.

Many people spend years hopping from one diet to another but are still confused about what or how much to eat. Add to this the pressure of modern living, being short of time and the confidence to cook, as well as being surrounded by tempting and readily accessible food, and it's little wonder we find it so hard not to put on weight. There isn't a magic solution, but you can take more control by learning more about what and how much to eat and starting to incorporate more activity into your life.

This chapter explains the background to the diet, giving you guidance about the food groups that will be part of your eating plans.

This chapter has several sections:

- **The key to weight-loss success** outlines the principles of energy balance.
- **What can I eat?** takes you through the food-group system, explaining the importance of each group and providing you with useful tips for your diet.
- **Your diet goal** provides a breakdown of the calories and fat that you may have at each meal.
- **Your meal blueprints** helps you to plan healthy, balanced meals by giving you a clear guide of what to include each mealtime.

- **Food and your mind** helps you to identity why you eat and provides a few tips to keep you motivated.

The Key to Weight-loss Success

Successful weight loss is about losing weight *and* keeping it off. To do this you need to understand how to eat and live healthily, not only while you are in your weight-loss phase, but beyond it, too. You also need to understand your own triggers to eating so that you can recognize when you are hungry, and when you are eating just because you are bored. More on this at the end of the chapter, but first some nutrition basics.

The Energy-balance Equation

Food and drink provide us with energy, which is measured in kilocalories, normally shortened to calories, or sometimes in joules and kilojoules. Our bodies use energy in a host of different ways: keeping our bodies ticking over – even digesting food needs calories; for maintenance and growth and the repair of our tissues and organs. We gain weight when we consume more energy (calories) than we use up, so in order to lose weight we need to consume fewer calories or use up more.

The healthiest way to lose weight is to use up more calories *as well as* consuming fewer. This is because:

- becoming more active is great for your health now and in the long term
- if you only cut down on food you run the risk of cutting out vital vitamins and minerals
- being active releases feel-good hormones, which help sustain your efforts and make you feel better
- you will improve your muscle tone
- studies have found that people who increase their activity as part of a diet maintain their weight-loss success for longer than those who only cut back on calories
- you are likely to lose weight faster.

Chapter 7 provides information on how to incorporate more activity into your daily life.

What Can I Eat?

This diet follows recommended nutrition principles for a healthier diet. That is, it encourages you to eat a balanced diet, eating foods from all the main food groups, control your calories through portion size and reduce fat intake, and also be more active.

This may not sound like rocket science. It isn't. The diet is designed so that:

1. you achieve effective, gradual weight loss
2. you lose weight by eating 'normal', not 'diet' foods
3. you learn to take control of your eating by understanding more about foods and nutrition.

Alongside the diet you are encouraged to become more active and also to spend some time looking at the triggers that may make you eat when you are not hungry. Whole books have been written on the motivational side of eating and slimming, and it is not within the scope of this book to provide more than a thumbnail sketch with some practical hints and pointers to help you.

To start off with, you need to look at what a healthy, balanced diet really is so you can begin to make better choices from now on.

What Is a Healthy Balanced Diet?

A healthy, balanced diet contains the right amount and mix of nutrients and energy for your individual needs. Not too much and not too little – a sort of Goldilocks principle.

That sounds all fine and dandy, but who knows exactly how much energy you need or which particular vitamins and minerals you need the most? Few people do, and even then it will vary week by week. So we need a way of showing what this may be for an average healthy person.

There are different ways this can be done. Sometimes a pyramid of food and drink is used, or a basket depicting a range of food groups. The UK model is called the Eatwell Plate and represents the type and amount of different foods that should form part of a healthy diet.

The idea is to show you the relative proportion of food groups you need to eat as part of a healthy diet. There are five groups:

The eatwell plate

Use the eatwell plate to help you get the balance right. It shows how
much of what you eat should come from each food group

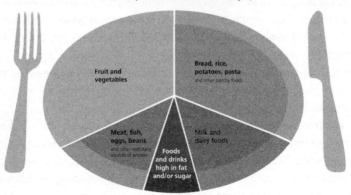

1. Fruit and vegetables
2. Bread, rice, potatoes, pasta and other starchy foods
3. Milk and dairy foods
4. Meat, fish, eggs, beans and other non-dairy sources of protein
5. Foods and drinks high in fat and/or sugar

If we all managed to eat these types of foods in suitable portions *and* were sufficiently active, we'd all have a healthy, balanced diet and be more likely to be a
healthy weight. Unfortunately, most of us eat more of one group than another,
especially the fatty and sugary foods group, and not enough of the fruit and
vegetables group, so we end up with a poorly balanced diet, which can lead
to overweight.

Let's take a closer look at each food group and how it fits into your weight-
loss diet.

Fruit and Vegetables

Fruit and vegetables are a really important part of any diet, as they provide a
wide range of different vitamins, minerals and important plant substances. Each
vegetable and fruit contains different amounts and types of these, so it is best
to include as many different fruit and vegetables as you can. Eating a range of
differently coloured fruit and vegetables each day is a good way to ensure you

have a mixture of these essentials. For example, carrots, sweet potato, mango and pawpaw (orange) are rich in vitamin A, while vegetables such as spinach and cabbage (dark green) provide vitamin K. Tomatoes, strawberries and peppers (red) are particularly rich in vitamin C, as too are orange and yellow citrus fruits.

Fruit and vegetables contain a high proportion of water compared to the amount of calories they provide. This means they have a low energy density, which is good news for dieters, as along with their general bulkiness they are great for filling you up without adding lots of calories or fat (with the exception of avocados).

An often overlooked dietary essential is fibre, which is found in all plant foods. Fibre is the term used for many different compounds, and each has its own beneficial functions in the body. Keeping your bowel habits regular relies on insoluble fibre. Soluble fibre, meanwhile, increases feelings of fullness and also has a positive influence on your blood cholesterol levels.

You should be aiming for at least five portions of fruit and vegetables each day. If you are uncertain as to what a portion is, have a look at Chapter 9 – but don't forget that juice only counts once a day, and potatoes don't count as vegetables. Also – to help you see that getting your five a day doesn't have to be difficult – the menu plans in Chapter 3 all include at least five portions of fruit and vegetables.

Bread, Rice, Potatoes, Pasta and Other Starchy Foods

This category also includes breakfast cereals, oats and other grains. Starchy carbohydrates should be the most important source of calories in your diet. Starches are a type of carbohydrate that provide energy, and it is important to eat a starchy food at every meal, including some wholegrain versions as these give you additional fibre, minerals such as iron and calcium and B vitamins.

Starchy foods, especially those that are wholegrain, can be filling and are much less energy-dense than fat or oil. One gram of carbohydrate provides less than half the calories per gram compared to fats such as butter and oil.

You may have heard of foods with a high or low 'GI' or glycaemic index. Foods with a low GI help regulate your blood sugar so you don't have surges of sugars in your blood after you've eaten, followed by a trough that leaves you feeling ravenous. These fluctuations are unhealthy and are thought to reduce the efficiency of the hormone insulin that controls your blood sugar. In the long term this can lead to diabetes. Foods with a high GI cause a sharp rise in your blood sugar, while those with a low GI cause a more gradual rise that is then prolonged. Having foods with a low GI helps you feel fuller for longer.

This diet encourages the use of lower-GI foods, and Chapter 9 provides nutrition and GI information on some commonly eaten foods. You may also find more information on the internet – and look for GI labels on some foods in supermarkets.

This is not a low-carbohydrate diet. Some people have great weight-loss results through cutting out carbohydrates, but for lifelong healthy eating this important food group provides essential nutrients and fibre.

Milk and Dairy Foods

Foods such as milk, yogurt and cheese (or the fortified soya alternatives) are essential for the calcium and vitamin B2 (riboflavin) they supply. Dairy products tend to contain a relatively high percentage of fat and saturated fat, but by choosing reduced-fat versions you will be able to meet your fat targets.

If you choose skimmed or semi-skimmed milk, reduced-fat yogurt and cheese, you will cut back on calories from fat and saturates but not on essential calcium or riboflavin.

You don't have to use fat-free dairy products when on the diet if you follow the recipes and menu plans, as the diet allows for about 30 per cent of your calories to come from fat. This means you don't lose out on vitamins A and D, which are important fat-soluble vitamins, found in milk and cheese.

Meat, Fish, Eggs, Beans and Other Non-dairy Sources of Protein

This group also includes poultry, lentils, soya, tofu and vegetarian alternatives. We need surprisingly little of these foods – just a couple of small portions a day – and as some of these foods can be high in fat it is important to choose them carefully. Meat should be lean, with visible fat removed and skin trimmed from poultry. How these foods are cooked will also influence their fat content, so use fat-free or low-fat cooking methods such as grilling, baking, steaming, poaching and braising.

It is important to include plenty of fish in your diet, at least two portions a week. You can still include one portion of oily fish such as salmon or tuna in your diet by eating a small portion, making sure it fits within your fat target. Oily fish is one of the very few sources of dietary vitamin D, and it also contains omega-3 fatty acids, which have a wide range of health benefits. White fish is naturally low in fat and a great part of any weight-loss diet.

Beans, lentils and peas are low in fat and high in fibre, which makes them ideal for your diet. You will find that you also eat eggs on the diet, probably just one per meal as egg yolk contains fat but is also a source of iron and vitamin A.

Nuts provide healthy unsaturated fats, and small quantities can be used in your diet if you weigh them out. They are a great addition to low-fat breakfast cereals. See Chapter 9 to make sure you only eat quantities that are consistent with your targets.

Foods and Drinks High in Fat and/or Sugar

These are, for most of us, our favourite foods – but these really are the ones we need the least, nutritionally. These foods include cakes, pastries, fried foods, chocolates, confectionery, biscuits, ice cream, mayonnaises, sauces and dressings. Drinks such as squashes, carbonated sweetened drinks and hot chocolate are high in sugars.

Butter and creams, oils and fat spreads of all types are included in this group because of their fat content. Fat contains more than twice the calories per gram compared with carbohydrates or protein. That is, they are very energy-dense, so by reducing the amount of fat in your diet you will decrease calories fast. However, some oils and vegetable fats contain beneficial unsaturated oils and vitamin E, so can be eaten in small quantities if you carefully measure them out.

The diet doesn't ban foods high in fat and sugar from your diet, as they do add variety and enjoyment. Banning something only makes it more attractive. There are some considerations you must bear in mind, however.

- Only eat fatty and sugary foods once you have had a balanced meal so are feeling fairly full.
- Ask yourself *why* you want to eat this food – see page 28 for some help.
- Make sure you know how many calories and grams of fat a portion contains. If it fits in your plan, then stick to the one item.
- Measure or weigh everything.

More on Fats

When you are on the diet you will be focusing on a total number of grams of fat you can eat. However, it is also important to consider what *sort* of fats you are eating.

Fat is found in many foods, and we tend to classify them into those that are said to be *saturated* and those that are *unsaturated*.

Put very simply, saturated fats increase your blood cholesterol levels, which can lead to your arteries becoming blocked. This increases your risk of developing heart disease. Saturated fats are found mostly in animal foods such as butter, ghee, lard, cream, cheese and meat, though certain plant foods such as coconut are also high in saturates.

Unsaturated fats can have a beneficial effect on your blood cholesterol and don't increase your risk of heart disease. There are many different types of unsaturated fats, from monounsaturates, which are found in olive and rapeseed oils and spreads made from them, to polyunsaturates, which are found in sunflower, nut, seed and fish oils. Omega-3 fatty acids are part of the group of polyunsaturates and are known to be beneficial for heart health as well as having other important health benefits.

Hydrogenated fats (or trans fats) are made when liquid oils are made into solid fats. Trans fats have been found to have a damaging effect on the body. In the UK, food manufacturers have removed almost all hydrogenated fats from foods, and foods must be labelled if they contain them.

Fluids

Having plenty of water in the diet is essential for your metabolism, not just to stop you feeling thirsty. Aim to drink at least 1.5 to 2 litres of water a day (this is about 6–8 glasses). You may include low-calorie flavoured drinks or fruit or herb teas in this. If you drink a lot of tea and coffee you should drink plenty of water as well, as tea and coffee are both slightly diuretic (cause you to excrete more water). Beware of the calories found in juices, smoothies and coffees such as lattes and cappuccinos. (See Chapter 5 for more about this.)

Lastly – A Note on Salt

A healthy diet needn't contain added salt unless you are very active or have been told to do so by your doctor. Having a diet high in salt increases your risk of high blood pressure and stroke, and by cutting down on salt you are protecting yourself. We should all be aiming to have no more than 6g of salt per day.

Many foods have salt added during manufacture or processing. Ham, bacon, salami and other cured meats are all high in salt, as are smoked fish, hard cheeses, pickles, chutneys, olives, soups and sauces, crisps and savoury snacks. Even foods that don't taste salty include some, such as bread, breakfast cereals and many baked goods.

The recipes in this book do not contain added salt, and if stock is used it is a reduced-salt variety. Each recipe includes the amount of salt per portion so you can monitor your salt intake. If you do like to add salt to food, add it at the table so not all the family has to have it, and always taste food *before* adding it. Try to cut down gradually – you can add a little bit less each time and will not notice the difference.

Your Diet Goal

In Chapter 1 you read about how to set your fat and calorie targets, so by now you will have chosen the targets that fit you best.

Amount of calories you can eat per day	Maximum amount of Fat allowed per meal	Maximum amount of Fat allowed per snack
1200	12g	3g
1400	15g	3g
1600	17g	3g
1800	19g	3g

Planning Your Meals

Based on the healthy, balanced diet model described previously, you can choose whether:

- to follow the suggested meal plans in the book (Chapter 3)
- to use the recipes in Chapter 4 to make up your own daily menus
- to buy ready-made foods that fit your targets with ideas from chapters 6 and 9.

You may of course do a combination of these depending on your circumstances and mood. Whatever you do, write a daily food diary.

The table below is a guide to help you plan your meals. It shows the recommended amount of calories (kcal) and fat for each meal occasion, including one or more snacks.

	1200kcal		1400kcal		1600kcal		1800kcal	
	kcal	Fat g	kcal	Fat g	kcal	Fat g	kcal	Fat g
Breakfast	300	<12	350	<15	400	<17	450	<19
Lunch	350	<12	400	<15	500	<17	550	<19
Dinner	400	<12	500	<15	550	<17	650	<19
Snack	150	<3	150	<3	150	<3	150	<3

Your Meal Blueprints

These blueprints provide the basics to help you plan healthy meals.

Breakfast Blueprint

1. A piece of fruit or some vegetables or a glass (250ml maximum) of unsweetened fruit juice or smoothie
2. A starchy food such as bread, rolls or crackers, ideally wholemeal or granary, or a bowl of breakfast cereal, muesli or porridge
3. A low-fat, preferably unsaturated spread to accompany the starchy foods, and/or a teaspoon of jam or marmalade

4. A measured amount of skimmed or semi-skimmed milk to have with your cereal and morning drink
5. A glass of water
6. You may also be able to include some other foods depending on which programme you are following

Have a look at Chapter 9 for fat and calorie guidance.

- A boiled or poached egg or grilled fat-trimmed back bacon with grilled tomato
- A slice or two of lean ham
- A small portion of cheese
- A few almonds or walnuts to add to your cereal
- A low-fat yogurt or probiotic drink

Midday Meal Blueprint

If you have your main meal in the evening then your lunch meal still needs to include a wide range of different foods to maximize the nutrients you get.

1. Include at least one, preferably two or more *fruit* or *vegetables*. For example, a mixed salad (for dressing, see note 5), a bowl of vegetable soup, an apple/pear/orange or a bowl of carrot and pepper sticks
2. A measured or weighed source of *starchy carbohydrate* such as bread, potato, pasta, rice etc. If you are buying a sandwich lunch, then have a look at the guide in Chapter 5
3. A source of protein – e.g. lean meat, fish, beans or lentils, an egg, or perhaps a small amount of cheese. Weigh these out so you recognize what a suitable portion looks like
4. A glass of water
5. Are you having any high-fat foods such as spreads or dressings? If you haven't reached your fat target, and can include them, make sure to measure them out
6. Can you add a low-fat yogurt or fromage frais to provide calcium if you have fat and calories to spare?

Evening Meal Blueprint

You may like to make this a two- or even three-course meal if your fat and calorie targets permit. Whatever the combination of foods you choose, make sure you follow the same guidelines as for lunch.

1. A minimum of one, preferably *two* portions of vegetables, plain, cooked or as salad
2. A *piece of fruit*, possibly as a starter or dessert
3. A measured portion of *protein-rich food* with associated low- or reduced-fat sauces or accompaniments
4. Measured *starchy foods* such as potatoes, sweet potatoes, brown rice, pasta, polenta, couscous or other grains cooked with minimal fat
5. A glass of water

Also consider
If you have calories and fat left over from your meal target, you may choose a glass of wine, a small dessert or a piece of chocolate. See Chapter 9 for some ideas.

Snacks Blueprint

Often the best snack is a piece of fruit along with a glass of water, but you can have a range of different types of snacks – provided they contain less than 3g of fat and are ideally 150kcal.

Remember that by choosing something that is low in GI then you are going to stay feeling fuller for longer.

Food and Your Mind

Anyone who has ever tried to lose weight knows how powerful your mind can be in constantly reminding you about how hungry you are, and making foods that are off-limits seem even more attractive than usual.

While is it not possible here to provide a comprehensive guide to the psychology of dieting, there are many tips that will help you on your way.

1. Set yourself a *realistic* goal, and write it down. Goals can be very personal – perhaps to wear a particular favourite outfit again, to return to your pre-pregnancy body weight, or to be ready for that holiday you are planning. Keep your goal with you so you can refer to it in moments of self-doubt.
2. Try to work out what role foods plays in your life – is it a comfort when you are unhappy or stressed? Do you eat when you are bored? By thinking this through you may be able to avoid falling into the trap of eating when you are not really hungry.
3. Plan your meals in advance, and make a note every day of what you ate and drank, your activity level and how you felt that day. Look back at it often to see if there are any links between your mood and what you did or ate. When you are feeling tempted to give up, focus on the good days and take strength from your previous successes.
4. Think about *how* you eat, and modify those things that are not helpful. For example if you tend to snack when you are preparing dinner, chop up carrot sticks in advance to munch on. If you are a habitual car-snacker, train yourself not to eat while in the car, perhaps drinking water instead. Have a proper meal time at the dining table rather than grazing while at the computer or watching TV. Developing these sorts of habits takes time but is worth the effort.
5. Be positive about yourself and what you are doing. Having a positive mental attitude can work wonders. Believe in yourself, and surround yourself with others who will support you.
6. When you are tempted, remind yourself how well you are doing, not listening to the negative voice within, and focus on the goal you have set yourself. If you do succumb to temptation, don't give up. Just keep going, focusing again on your goal.
7. Don't forget the psychological benefit of being active. Go for a 10-minute brisk walk rather than 10 minutes of munchies. Enlist family and friends to exercise with you, and make this a regular event.
8. Talk positively to people – including yourself – about what you are doing. This will help strengthen your willpower and remind you of the benefits of your diet rather than feeling it is all about giving up things.

Chapter 3

The Menu Plans

In this chapter you will find a range of different menu plans to help guide you through and beyond the time you are dieting. There are menu plans to fit the different calorie and fat bands of your diet. Included here are four weeks of daily menus for the 1400-calorie diet, the one that is most commonly followed. Additionally there is one menu plan per week for each of the 1200-, 1600- and 1800-calorie diets. These plans may also be useful if you are just starting out on the diet, or are coming to the end of your diet and want to maintain weight rather than lose it.

The menu plans can be used in several ways. When dieting, some people like to know exactly what they can eat down to the last lettuce leaf. If you are one of those people the menu plans are perfect, as they describe each meal and snack. They provide links to the recipes in Chapter 4 (the recipe name is in *italics*). If there is a meal you don't fancy, you can find a substitute by looking at Chapter 4, by searching for a ready-prepared option in Chapter 6 or by putting ingredients from Chapter 9 together.

Other people use menu plans for inspiration, gleaning ideas for meals but making up their own menus. If this is the way you like to diet, then you can easily find information to suit your calorie and fat targets by using chapters 4, 6 and 9. It is worth writing down your own menu plan so you can check that you keep within your fat and calorie targets.

A Reminder of the Fat and Calorie Targets

The table that follows shows you the maximum number of calories and grams of fat you can eat. The menu plans are worked out on a daily basis, so use the information in the first two columns. If you are making up your own meal plans, you will need to ensure that you keep to the fat targets for each meal or snack.

Amount of calories you can eat per day	Maximum amount of fat per day	Maximum amount of fat allowed per meal	Minimum amount of fat allowed per snack
1200	39	12g	3g
1400	48	15g	3g
1600	54	17g	3g
1800	60	19g	3g

Menu Plan Instructions

The table below suggests how you may break your daily fat and calorie allowance down.

	1200kcal		1400kcal		1600kcal		1800kcal	
	kcal	Fat g	kcal	Fat g	kcal	Fat g	kcal	Fat g
Breakfast	300	<12	350	<15	350	<16	500	<16
Lunch	350	<12	400	<15	400	<16	500	<16
Dinner	400	<12	500	<15	500	<16	500	<16
Snack	150	<3	150	<3	150	<3	150	<3
Snack	–	–	–	–	150	<3	150	<3

- Each day you should have 300ml skimmed milk (or non dairy equivalent) for cereals, drinks and in cooking. (This helps ensure you are having adequate calcium.) Measure it out at the start of the day, so you know how much you are using.
- Drink at least 1.5 litres (6 x250ml glasses) of water a day in addition to other drinks. You may have low calorie squashes and unsweetened herb or fruit teas in addition to tea and cofee, but do not forget to count in sugar or milk you are adding.
- Drinks such as juices, smoothies and alcoholic drinks all add calories so unless stated are not included in the menu plans.
- Make sure you measure everything out. The menu plans give weights and, where appropriate, household measures.
- Recipes from the book are shown in *italic* text. If you don't like the recipe, simply find another with similar fat and calories by looking at the charts at the end of Chapter 4, by choosing a ready made option from one of the supermarkets (see Chapter 6) or by using Chapter 9 to construct your own meal.

1400-calorie Diet

1400kcal, 48g fat per day
Week 1

Day 1

Breakfast	50g extra-fruit muesli; 125g low-fat fruit yogurt.
Mid-morning	1 medium banana.
Midday meal	1 (64g) wholemeal wrap; 2 tsp (10g) olive spread, 35g honey-roast salmon flakes, sliced cucumber; 1 apple.
Afternoon	Glass of milk from daily allowance.
Evening meal	1 portion *Fresh Pea and Ham Risotto*; salad of watercress and 4 cherry tomatoes; *Oranges with Fresh Dates and Honey Yogurt*.
Nutrition	**1400kcal, 32g fat and 5 portions of fruit and vegetables.**

Day 2

Breakfast	1 piece *Spelt and Walnut Scone Round*; 30g medium-fat soft cheese; 200ml glass orange juice.
Mid-morning	1 digestive biscuit.
Midday meal	1 portion *Watercress Soup* with 25g grated reduced-fat cheddar; granary roll thinly spread with 1 tsp (5g) polyunsaturated spread and 1 slice lean ham; 1 medium pear.
Afternoon	80g grapes.
Evening meal	*Hot Garlicky King Prawn Salad*; 1 pot crème caramel with 100g strawberries topped with 1 tbsp (30g) Greek yogurt.
Nutrition	**1378kcal, 42g fat and 5 portions of fruit and vegetables.**

Day 3

Breakfast	1 boiled egg; 2 slices wholemeal toast with 2 tsp (10g) olive spread; 150g melon cubes.
Mid-morning	Glass of milk from daily allowance.
Midday meal	Subway 6-inch Sub Steak and cheese; 250ml pressed apple juice.
Afternoon	40g carrot sticks with 2 breadsticks.
Evening meal	1 portion *Home-made Burgers with Spicy Potato Wedges* with 1 portion *Raspberry Salsa*; 50g salad leaves; large slice (100g) fresh pineapple.
Nutrition	**1400kcal, 38.5g fat and 5 portions of fruit and vegetables.**

Day 4

Breakfast	30g branflakes with 3 chopped walnut halves and 30g (1 tbsp) sultanas; skimmed milk from daily allowance.
Mid-morning	150g carton low-fat fruit yogurt.
Midday meal	300ml Carrot and coriander soup (e.g. M&S); ciabatta roll (70g) spread with 2 tsp olive spread (10g); 25g premium ham; 1 apple.
Afternoon	200ml pressed unsweetened apple juice.
Evening meal	1 portion *Spicy Lamb* with 40g (dry weight) basmati rice; 50g plain naan bread; *Raita* made with 25g grated cucumber and 1 tbsp (35g) low-fat yogurt, black pepper.
Nutrition	**1416kcal, 37.4g fat and 5 portions of fruit and vegetables.**

Day 5

Breakfast	2 slices (72g) granary toast with 2 tsp (10g) olive spread and marmalade; 250ml mango and passion fruit smoothie.
Mid-morning	Hot-chocolate drink made from 18g reduced-fat chocolate powder and milk from allowance.
Midday meal	½ Pizza Express La Reine (141g) with salad of 4 cherry tomatoes, handful (40g) leaves and 1 tbsp fat-free dressing.
Afternoon	80g fresh raspberries or other seasonal fruit.
Evening meal	1 portion *Cherry Tomato and Smoked Haddock Kedgeree*; small pot (45g) chocolate mousse (e.g. M&S).
Nutrition	**1415kcal, 37.4g fat and 5 portions of fruit and vegetables.**

Day 6

Breakfast	Grapefruit, either half, or 120g drained, canned in juice; porridge using 45g oats, milk from allowance; top with 1 tbsp (20g) honey and 15g toasted almonds.
Mid-morning	1 medium orange or 2 clementines.
Midday meal	Salad made with 30g lettuce, 1 medium tomato, 4 radishes, 1 nectarine and 54g (7) mozzarella pearls (tiny balls); 1 tbsp (15g) balsamic glaze; ½ baguette (67g).
Afternoon	Glass of milk from allowance.
Evening meal	90g pasta – e.g. fusilli tricolore with *Pasta Sauce with Mediterranean Vegetables*; 1 dsp (10g) grated parmesan.
Nutrition	**1392kcal, 36.3g fat and 6 portions of fruit and vegetables.**

Day 7

Breakfast	40g Crunchy oat cereal with honey and almond with milk from allowance; 200ml glass unsweetened orange juice.
Mid-morning	80g grapes.
Midday meal	Panini roll (85g) filled with 30g slice ham, 35g grated mozzarella and 1 tsp (5g) caramelized onion chutney;1 pear.
Afternoon	Glass of milk from allowance.
Evening meal	100g portion of *Citrus Couscous*; 130g roasted chicken without skin; 90g green beans; small scoop (75g) chocolate ice cream.
Nutrition	**1414kcal, 38g fat and 5 portions of fruit and vegetables.**

Also included: each day you may have 300ml skimmed milk (or non-dairy equivalent) for cereals and drinks. Drink at least 1.5 litres (6 x 250ml glasses) of water a day. Drinks such as juices, smoothies, alcohol etc. are not included unless stated.

1400-calorie Diet

Day 1

Breakfast	1 large boiled egg with 2 crumpets spread with 2 tsp (10g) olive spread and scraping yeast extract; 1 large satsuma.
Mid-morning	1 *Maple and Raisin Drop Scone* spread with 15g (1 level tbsp) extra-light soft cheese.
Midday meal	1 portion *Pea Soup with Pesto Croute*; 1 slice wholemeal bread with 1 tsp (5g) olive spread; 1 pear.
Afternoon	Glass of milk from allowance.
Evening meal	1 portion *Turkey Steak with Crumb and Sundried Tomato Topping*; 120g boiled new potatoes; 120g fresh fruit salad with 1 scoop (60g) reduced-fat ice cream.
Nutrition	**1405kcal, 42g fat and 5 to 6 portions of fruit and vegetables.**

Day 2

Breakfast	150g carton low-fat fruit yogurt with 100g fresh berries and 1 tbsp (16g) sunflower seeds.
Mid-morning	Glass of milk from allowance.
Midday meal	*Smoked Trout Sandwich with Horseradish and Lamb's Lettuce* (or retail equivalent, providing about 310kcal and 7.7g fat); 25g bag low-fat crisps e.g Walkers Baked; 1 medium apple.
Afternoon	30g sultanas or other dried fruit.
Evening meal	1 portion *Simple Cod Bake*; 175g potatoes mashed with 2 tsp (10g) olive spread and milk from allowance; 100g peas.
Nutrition	**1400kcal, 33.6g fat and 6 portions of fruit and vegetables.**

Day 3

Breakfast	Half a grapefruit; 50g bowl extra-fruit muesli with 10 (20g) almonds, chopped with milk from allowance.
Mid-morning	1 cereal bar (e.g. Cheerios bar).
Midday meal	1 portion *Curried Parsnip and Apple Soup*; 70g piece of baguette with 25g brie and half a red pepper cut into strips.
Afternoon	Glass of milk from allowance.
Evening meal	75g pasta shapes with 1 portion *Pasta Sauce with Artichokes and Peppers*; 15g (1 heaped tbsp) grated parmesan; side salad of leaves, cucumber and grated carrot; 150g slice melon with 1 tsp chopped stem ginger in syrup.
Nutrition	**1405kcal, 43.5g fat and 6 portions of fruit and vegetables.**

Day 4

Breakfast	1 *Cheese and Apple Scone* with 2 tsp (10g) olive spread and 1 medium apple, sliced.
Mid-morning	200ml mango and passion fruit smoothie.
Midday meal	*Bruschetta with Mozzarella, Basil and Tomatoes*; 80g strawberries topped with 1 level tbsp (15g) half-fat sour cream and 1 tsp sugar.
Afternoon	1 carrot cut into batons.
Evening meal	1 portion *Sunflower Seed-coated Chicken with Yogurt Herb Salad*; 50g warmed ciabatta drizzled with 1 tsp olive oil; 1 portion *Autumn Fruit Salad*.
Nutrition	**1396kcal, 39.1g fat and 7 portions of fruit and vegetables.**

Day 5

Breakfast	1 portion *Four-grain Porridge with Apricots* with 14g (4 halves) walnut halves, chopped, and 1 tsp (8g) runny honey.
Mid-morning	Glass of milk from allowance.
Midday meal	Sandwich – e.g *Piquant Egg and Watercress* (or bought equivalent – 365kcal and 11.3g fat).
Afternoon	200ml unsweetened orange juice.
Evening meal	1 portion *Monkfish and Prawn Kebabs* with 1 portion *Coconut Rice*; 90g steamed green beans; 1 portion *Bramley and Mango Brûlée*.
Nutrition	**1394kcal, 35.6g fat and 5 portions of fruit and vegetables.**

Day 6

Breakfast	2 *Buttermilk Pancakes* with 3 tsp maple syrup, 1 chopped banana and 1 rounded tbsp half-fat sour cream.
Mid-morning	Glass of milk from allowance.
Midday meal	1 portion *Hot Garlicky King Prawn Salad*; 1 sultana cookie (M&S) or equivalent.
Afternoon	80g grapes.
Evening meal	1 portion *Chinese-style Soup with Tiny Pork Balls*; 1 portion *Steak and Mangetout Stir-fry*.
Nutrition	**1381kcal, 33.6g fat and 5 portions of fruit and vegetables.**

Day 7

Breakfast	2 slices lean back bacon, grilled with 1 tomato; 2 small slices (50g) wholemeal bread, toasted and spread with 2 tsp (10g) olive spread.
Mid-morning	200ml orange or other unsweetened juice.
Midday meal	*Mexican Chicken in Chocolate* with 1 portion *Warm Potato Salad with Herbs*; 1 serving *Sweetcorn Salsa* and 90g steamed green beans.
Afternoon	150g pot virtually fat-free yogurt.
Evening meal	1 portion *Creamy Cherry Tomato Soup*; 1 serving *Apple and Cranberry Crisp.*
Nutrition	**1410kcal, 39g fat and 6 portions of fruit and vegetables.**

Also included: each day you may have 300ml skimmed milk (or non-dairy equivalent) for cereals and drinks. Drink at least 1.5 litres (6 x 250ml glasses) of water a day. Drinks such as juices, smoothies, alcohol etc. are not included unless stated.

1400-calorie Diet

Day 1

Breakfast	50g muesli with 1 tbsp (16g) sunflower seeds and 125g pot plain low-fat yogurt.
Mid-morning	1 medium satsuma.
Midday meal	1 portion *Asparagus and Egg Salad with Baby New Potatoes*; 2 medium plums.
Afternoon	1 digestive biscuit.
Evening meal	1 portion *Spaghetti with Chilli Prawns*; 1 portion *Fruits of the Forest Soufflé*.
Nutrition	**1400kcal, 40.7g fat and 5 portions of fruit and vegetables.**

Day 2

Breakfast	50g oatcakes spread with 45g (1 heaped tbsp) medium-fat soft cheese; 1 pear cut into slices.
Mid-morning	Cereal bar such as Fruit and Fibre.
Midday meal	1 *Warm Wrap with Refried Beans, Avocado and Peppers*, or shop-bought equivalent (390kcal and 13.8g fat); 80g grapes.
Afternoon	Glass of milk from allowance.
Evening meal	Omelette: 1 egg whisked with 1 egg white, cooked in 1 tsp olive oil, filled with wilted spinach and 4 slices wafer-thin lean ham; 120g (6 baby) new potatoes and 6 cherry tomatoes; 1 portion *Baked Peaches with Amaretti Filling* with 1 level tbsp reduced-fat crème fraîche.
Nutrition	**1380kcal, 44.7g fat and 6 portions of fruit and vegetables.**

Day 3

Breakfast	*Greek Yogurt with Berries and Walnuts.*
Mid-morning	1 small ginger biscuit. 200ml glass apple juice.
Midday meal	Bought soup, e.g. 300ml carrot and coriander, with 50g crusty roll spread with 2 tsp olive spread, and filled with 4 wafer-thin slices lean ham; 25g bag baked crisps.
Afternoon	Glass of milk from allowance.
Evening meal	130g portion grilled or roasted chicken, without skin; 1 portion *Ratatouille*; 50g couscous cooked according to the packet instructions with 1 tsp (5g) toasted pinenuts.
Nutrition	**1400kcal, 39g fat and 5 to 6 portions of fruit and vegetables.**

Day 4

Breakfast	Boiled egg with 1 wholemeal muffin spread with 2 tsp (10g) olive spread; 120g portion grapefruit canned in juice.
Mid-morning	1 large kiwi fruit (80g).
Midday meal	*Smoked Mackerel with Carrot and Currant Salad*; 200ml mango, passion fruit and pineapple smoothie.
Afternoon	Glass of milk from allowance.
Evening meal	1 portion *Chilli con Carne* with 40g (dry weight) basmati rice; 40g salad leaves with 1 tbsp *Yogurt and Herb Dressing*; 1 scoop (60g) low-fat ice cream.
Nutrition	**1380kcal, 42.4g fat and 6 portions of fruit and vegetables.**

Day 5

Breakfast	2 medium slices wholemeal bread thinly spread with peanut butter (24g); 1 small orange.
Mid-morning	1 *Maple and Raisin Drop Scone* spread with 1 tsp lemon curd.
Midday meal	*Pear and Feta Salad* with 40g French bread.
Afternoon	Glass of milk from allowance.
Evening meal	1 portion *Duck with Water Chestnuts and Noodles*; 100g mixed berries.
Nutrition	**1395kcal, 38.2g fat and 6 portions of fruit and vegetables.**

Day 6

Breakfast	1 poached egg on 1 slice granary bread lightly spread with 1 tsp (5g) olive spread; 1 slice (150g) melon.
Mid-morning	150g pot fat-free Greek yogurt with 2 tsp runny honey.
Midday meal	1 *Bacon- and Sweetcorn-stuffed Sweet Potato*; 100g grapes.
Afternoon	1 digestive biscuit.
Evening meal	1 portion *Pork Chop in Citrus Sauce*; 120g baby new potatoes; 90g mangetout; 1 portion *Bramley and Mango Brûlée*.
Nutrition	**1409kcal, 38g fat and 5 portions of fruit and vegetables.**

Day 7

Breakfast	*Breakfast Smoothie*; 2 rashers grilled lean back bacon served on 1 slice granary bread spread with 1 level tbsp tomato ketchup.
Mid-morning	1 *Chocolate and Cheerios Fruit Snack*.
Midday meal	*Tuna and Edamame Salad with Avocado and Green Beans* with *Chilli and Coriander Dressing*.
Afternoon	Glass of milk from allowance.
Evening meal	1 portion *Beef with Sweet Chestnuts* with 1 small (100g) baked potato with 1 rounded tbsp (35g) half-fat sour cream; 95g lightly boiled cabbage.
Nutrition	**1400kcal, 41g fat and 5 portions of fruit and vegetables.**

Also included: each day you may have 300ml skimmed milk (or non-dairy equivalent) for cereals and drinks. Drink at least 1.5 litres (6 x 250ml glasses) of water a day. Drinks such as juices, smoothies, alcohol etc. are not included unless stated.

1400-calorie Diet

1400kcal, 48g fat per day
Week 4

Day 1

Breakfast	1 portion *Breakfast Compote*; 1 (60g) plain croissant.
Mid-morning	Glass of milk from daily allowance.
Midday meal	1 portion *Cauliflower and Almond Soup* (or similar 125kcal and 4.5g fat per portion); 1 slice (35g) crusty white bread topped with 30g medium fat (15% fat) soft cheese and 50g sliced cucumber; 1 (55g) ready-to-eat fig.
Afternoon	1 small banana.
Evening meal	1 plaice fillet, grilled, served with 1 tsp (5g) butter; 1 portion *Polenta with Parmesan and Shallots*; 80g petits pois.
Nutrition	**1408kcal, 36.1g fat and 6 portions of fruit and vegetables.**

Day 2

Breakfast	Half a grapefruit; 1 boiled egg with 1 wholemeal muffin spread with 2 tsp (10g) olive spread.
Mid-morning	1 *Apricot and Coconut Muffin*.
Midday meal	1 portion *Pearl Barley and Pomegranate Salad* with 50g feta cheese and 40g salad leaves.
Afternoon	1 medium pear.
Evening meal	1 portion *Minty Chicken with Leek*; *Crushed New Potatoes with Herbs and Olive Oil*; 90g steamed green beans; 1 portion *Rice Pudding with Cardamom and Maple Syrup*.
Nutrition	**1380kcal, 42g fat and 5 portions of fruit and vegetables.**

Day 3

Breakfast	1 fruit teacake (73g) toasted and spread with 2 tsp (10g) olive spread; hot chocolate made with 3 tsp drinking chocolate powder and milk from allowance.
Mid-morning	2 small satsumas.
Midday meal	1 portion *Pumpkin Soup* with 1 multiseed tortilla wrap spread with quarter-pot (50g) extra-light soft cheese and 30g rocket; 1 medium apple.
Afternoon	2 plums.
Evening meal	1 portion *Pork Patties* with 1 tbsp *Spicy Harissa Dressing*; 30g (dry weight) bulghar wheat and 6 baby plum tomatoes; 2 scoops (120g) mango sorbet.
Nutrition	**1380kcal, 35.3g fat and 5 portions of fruit and vegetables.**

Day 4

Breakfast	50g crunchy oat and honey cereal, with 1 small chopped banana with milk from daily allowance.
Mid-morning	125g pot low-fat fruit yogurt.
Midday meal	1 *Smoked Trout Sandwich with Horseradish* or retail equivalent (310kcal and 7.7g fat).
Afternoon	1 digestive biscuit.
Evening meal	1 portion *Pasta, Pesto and Chicken Salad*; 1 portion *Baked Plums with Port* with 1 level tbsp (15g) half-fat crème fraîche.
Nutrition	**1390kcal, 33.5g fat and 5 portions of fruit and vegetables.**

Day 5

Breakfast	1 portion *Grapefruit Salad with Toasted Almonds*; 1 *Buttermilk Pancake* with 1 tsp maple syrup.
Mid-morning	1 square *Chocolate Mallow Crispies*.
Midday meal	1 wholemeal pitta filled with 1 portion *Home-made Houmous* and 2 tbsp (40g) raw bean sprouts; 1 (25g) crunchy cereal bar.
Afternoon	Glass of milk from daily allowance.
Evening meal	1 portion *Spinach and Mushroom Pasta Bake*; 1 portion *Autumn Fruit Salad*.
Nutrition	**1415kcal, 44g fat and 5 portions of fruit and vegetables.**

Day 6

Breakfast	*Greek Yogurt with Berries and Walnuts*; 200ml unsweetened orange juice.
Mid-morning	1 *Chocolate and Cheerios Fruit Snack*.
Midday meal	1 portion *Bacon and Sweetcorn Chowder*; 1 kiwi fruit.
Afternoon	Glass of milk from daily allowance.
Evening meal	1 portion *Chicken with Cajun Spices and Chickpeas*; 1 portion *Apricot and Ginger Rice*; 85g green beans, steamed.
Nutrition	**1392kcal, 42.1g fat and 5 portions of fruit and vegetables.**

Day 7

Breakfast	2 *Buttermilk Pancakes* with 150g fruits of the forest stewed with 2 tsp sugar; 1 rounded tbsp (40g) half-fat crème fraîche.
Mid-morning	Glass of milk from daily allowance.
Midday meal	1 portion *Lamb and Apricot Tagine*; 1 portion *Watercress and Orange Salad*.
Afternoon	Glass of water.
Evening meal	*Tuna and Olive Black Bulghar Wheat Salad*; 2 small chocolates.
Nutrition	**1385kcal, 36.5g fat and 5 portions of fruit and vegetables.**

Also included: each day you may have 300ml skimmed milk (or non-dairy equivalent) for cereals and drinks. Drink at least 1.5 litres (6 x 250ml glasses) of water a day. Drinks such as juices, smoothies, alcohol etc. are not included unless stated.

1200-calorie Diet

1200kcal, 39g fat per day

Day 1

Breakfast	*Breakfast Smoothie*; 30g branflakes and 25 (1 tbsp) sultanas with skimmed milk from daily allowance.
Mid-morning	Glass of milk from allowance.
Midday meal	*Pea Soup with Pesto Croute,* 1 (50g) granary roll spread with 2 tsp (10g) <40% fat spread; 1 medium apple.
Afternoon	60g virtually fat-free fromage frais.
Evening meal	1 portion *Grilled Teriyaki Pork with Orange* with 1 portion *Warm Potato Salad with Herbs*; 50g wilted baby spinach leaves and 80g baby plum tomatoes; 1 ripe peach.
Nutrition	**1198kcal, 32g fat and 5 portions of fruit and vegetables.**

Day 2

Breakfast	2 slices (72g) granary bread toasted; lightly spread with olive spread (14g) and yeast extract (optional). 1 medium orange.
Mid-morning	60g virtually fat-free fromage frais.
Midday meal	Buy sandwich that provides about 280kcal and 8.5g fat (e.g. egg salad healthy option). Glass of milk from allowance.
Afternoon	80g grapes.
Evening meal	1 portion *Galettes with Spinach, Mushroom and Soft Goat's Cheese*; 150g slice melon with 1 tsp chopped stem ginger.
Nutrition	**1195kcal, 36.7g fat and 5 portions of fruit and vegetables.**

Day 3

Breakfast	1 portion *Grapefruit Salad with Toasted Almonds.*
Mid-morning	Glass of milk from allowance.
Midday meal	3 mini pitta bread (90g) with 1 portion *Smoked Trout Paté* and 2 celery sticks or 70g cucumber.
Afternoon	125g low-fat fruit yogurt.
Evening meal	1 portion *Moussaka* with 120g boiled new potatoes, 40g leaf salad and 4 (60g) cherry tomatoes.
Nutrition	**1215kcal, 39g fat and 5 portions of fruit and vegetables.**

Day 4

Breakfast	50g extra-fruit muesli with 6 (13g) chopped almonds; skimmed milk from allowance.
Mid-morning	Glass of milk from allowance.
Midday meal	300ml carrot and coriander soup (bought) with 30g slice of ciabatta and 25g piece of reduced-fat Edam or similar cheese.
Afternoon	200ml unsweetened orange juice.
Evening meal	1 portion *Tripoline with Lemon Mushrooms* and 1 portion *Watercress and Orange Salad.*
Nutrition	**1201kcal, 29g fat and 7 portions of fruit and vegetables.**

Day 5

Breakfast	1 egg scrambled with 25ml skimmed milk (from allowance) cooked in 1 tsp (5g) 40%-fat spread, served on 1 slice granary toast, with 80g grilled tomatoes; 1 additional slice granary toast spread with 1 tsp (5g) 40%-fat spread.
Mid-morning	40g ready-to-eat apricots.
Midday meal	*Chicken Tikka Pitta with Raita*; 160g chopped fresh fruit such as mango, pineapple and kiwi.
Afternoon	Milky coffee or glass of milk, both from allowance.
Evening meal	1 portion *Baked Plaice with Warm Lentil Salad* served with 1 portion *Crushed New Potatoes with Herbs and Olive Oil* and 90g steamed green beans.
Nutrition	**1200kcal, 33.1g fat and 6 portions of fruit and vegetables.**

Day 6

Breakfast	1 portion *Four-grain Porridge with Apricots* with skimmed milk from allowance.
Mid-morning	1 large kiwi fruit (80g).
Midday meal	1 portion *Hot Garlicky King Prawn Salad*; glass of milk from daily allowance.
Afternoon	1 square *Chocolate and Cheerios Fruit Snack*.
Evening meal	1 portion *Three Bean Curry* with 1 portion *Potatoes with Mustard Seeds and Spinach*.
Nutrition	**1196kcal, 27.8g fat and 6 portions of fruit and vegetables.**

Day 7

Breakfast	Brunch of *Poached Egg Muffin with Spinach and Mushrooms*.
Mid-morning	—
Midday meal	1 portion *Coq au Vin* with 50g French bread and 90g green beans.
Afternoon	Chocolate milkshake made with 1 tbsp (15g) reduced-fat chocolate powder and milk from allowance.
Evening meal	1 portion *Bacon and Sweetcorn Chowder*; 1 clementine.
Nutrition	**1205kcal, 41.6g fat and 5 portions of fruit and vegetables.**

Also included: each day you may have 300ml skimmed milk (or non-dairy equivalent) for cereals and drinks. Drink at least 1.5 litres (6 x 250ml glasses) of water a day. Drinks such as juices, smoothies, alcohol etc. are not included unless stated.

1600-calorie Diet

1600kcal, 54g fat per day

Day 1

Breakfast	1 *Cheese and Apple Scone* lightly spread with 10g (2 tsp) olive spread; 150g pot low-fat fruit yogurt.
Mid-morning	1 pear, apple or orange.
Midday meal	*Ciabatta Roll with Pesto, Soft Cheese and Baby Spinach*; 30g bag baked crisps or equivalent.
Afternoon	1 *Apricot and Coconut Muffin*.
Evening meal	130g grilled skinless chicken breast served with 1 portion *Pomegranate Sauce,* 1 portion *Coconut Rice*, broccoli (85g) and sweetcorn (95g); 1 portion *Fruits of the Forest Mousse*.
Nutrition	**1598kcal, 49g fat and 5 portions of fruit and vegetables.**

Day 2

Breakfast	2 slices (72g) granary bread lightly spread with 2 tsp (10g) olive spread; 25g piece of brie and 1 medium pear.
Mid-morning	Glass of milk from daily allowance.
Midday meal	1 portion *Moroccan Chickpea and Fruit Soup*, 1 wholemeal tortilla wrap filled with 1 chopped hardboiled egg, 1 level tbsp reduced-fat mayonnise and 1 medium tomato, skinned and chopped, mixed together.
Afternoon	1 *Mincemeat and Plum Filo Pie*.
Evening meal	1 portion *Stuffed Butternut Squash* with 90g wilted spinach leaves; 1 portion *No-fat Eton Mess*.
Nutrition	**1608kcal, 52g fat and 7 portions of fruit and vegetables.**

Day 3

Breakfast	1 portion *Four-grain Porridge with Apricots* sprinkled with 1 tbsp toasted sunflower seeds.
Mid-morning	Glass of milk from daily allowance.
Midday meal	Low-fat soup, e.g. 1 portion *Carrot and Celery Soup,* with *Mozzarella and Ham Panini.*
Afternoon	250ml smoothie, e.g. summerfruit.
Evening meal	1 large portion *Lasagne*; side salad of leaves, peppers and 25g marinated olives.
Nutrition	**1605kcal, 48.3g fat and 6 portions of fruit and vegetables.**

Day 4

Breakfast	1 egg scrambled with 25ml skimmed milk (from allowance) cooked in 1 tsp (5g) 40%-fat spread, served on 1 slice granary toast, with 80g grilled tomatoes; 1 additional slice granary toast spread with 1 tsp (5g) 40%-fat spread; 200ml unsweetened orange juice.
Mid-morning	1 small chocolate chip cookie.
Midday meal	1 portion *Bruschetta with Mozzarella, Basil and Tomatoes*; 25g pack reduced-fat crisps.
Afternoon	1 medium apple.
Evening meal	1 portion *Citrus Couscous* with 1 portion *Beef Koftas with Tzatziki*; 90g steamed mangetout.
Nutrition	**1598kcal, 49g fat and 5 portions of fruit and vegetables.**

Day 5

Breakfast	*Greek Yogurt with Berries and Walnuts*; 200ml pineapple or other unsweetened juice.
Mid-morning	6 tiny (32g) amaretti biscuits.
Midday meal	1 portion *Asparagus and Egg Salad with Baby New Potatoes*; 1 portion *Rice Pudding with Cardamom and Maple Syrup*.
Afternoon	Glass of milk from daily allowance.
Evening meal	1 portion *Jambalaya*; 100g strawberries with 1 level tbsp half-fat crème fraîche.
Nutrition	**1600kcal, 44.6g fat and 5 portions of fruit and vegetables.**

Day 6

Breakfast	1 portion *Spelt and Walnut Scone Round* spread with 2 tsp (10g) olive spread and 1 heaped tsp (15g) jam; 120g drained canned grapefruit topped with 1 rounded tbsp low-fat yogurt.
Mid-morning	1 banana.
Midday meal	*Bacon- and Sweetcorn-stuffed Sweet Potato.*
Afternoon	Glass of milk from daily allowance.
Evening meal	1 portion *Lemony Salmon with Thyme Couscous and Onion Salad*; 175ml glass dry white wine; 1 portion *Fruits of the Forest Mousse*.
Nutrition	**1591kcal, 48.5g fat and 5 portions of fruit and vegetables.**

Day 7

Breakfast	2 *Buttermilk Pancakes* with 1 rounded tbsp half-fat crème fraîche and compote made by stewing 150g frozen summer fruits with 1 tbsp (15g) sugar.
Mid-morning	1 large satsuma.
Midday meal	1 portion *Pumpkin Soup* with 1 *Ham and Cheese Toastie*.
Afternoon	Glass of milk with 1 gingernut biscuit.
Evening meal	1 portion *Topside with Winter Vegetables*; 1 portion *Baked Peaches with Amaretti Filling* with 2 level tbsp (30g) half-fat crème fraîche.
Nutrition	**1600kcal, 48.5g fat and 6 portions of fruit and vegetables.**

Also included: each day you may have 300ml skimmed milk (or non-dairy equivalent) for cereals and drinks. Drink at least 1.5 litres (6 x 250ml glasses) of water a day. Drinks such as juices, smoothies, alcohol etc. are not included unless stated.

1800-calorie Diet

1800kcal, 60g fat per day

Day 1

Breakfast	30g Crunchy Nut Cornflakes with milk from allowance; 1 crumpet lightly spread with 1 tsp (5g) olive spread and 35g piece Edam cheese; 1 large satsuma or small orange.
Mid-morning	200ml apple juice and 1 square *Chocolate Mallow Crispies*.
Midday meal	1 portion *Watercress Soup*; 1 ham sandwich made with 2 slices granary bread, spread with 30g soft goat's cheese and 2 slices (24g) Parma ham, and 25g salad leaves.
Afternoon	1 medium apple, peach or pear.
Evening meal	1 portion *Greek Baked Chicken with Okra* with 175g new potatoes, 90g sugar snaps; 1 purchased pancake with juice of half a lemon, 1 chopped small banana and 1 tsp soft brown sugar.
Nutrition	**1803kcal, 50g fat and 6 to 7 portions of fruit and vegetables.**

Day 2

Breakfast	2 rashers (50g) lean back bacon, grilled with 2 medium tomatoes; 1 wholemeal muffin spread with 2 tsp (10g) olive spread; 200ml grapefruit juice.
Mid-morning	Glass of milk from allowance.
Midday meal	*Baked Potato with Curried Prawns*; 150g pot fat-free Greek yogurt, with 1 tsp (5g) runny honey and 10g chopped almonds.
Afternoon	200ml exotic fruit smoothie.
Evening meal	1 portion *Pork in Dijon Mustard Sauce with Leek Mash*, 85g steamed carrots and 85g steamed broccoli; 130g canned pears in juice, with 1 portion *Bitter Chocolate Sauce*.
Nutrition	**1798kcal, 46.6g fat and 7 portions of fruit and vegetables.**

Day 3

Breakfast	1 large egg, poached and served on 2 slices wholemeal toast lightly spread with 3 tsp (15g) olive spread; 110g stewed fruit (apricots/plums/ apples).
Mid-morning	1 piece *Chocolate and Cheerios Fruit Snack*.
Midday meal	1 portion *Creamy Cherry Tomato Soup* with 1 *Sundried Tomato and Black Olive Scone* with 2 tsp (10g) olive spread.
Afternoon	150g fat-free yogurt with 1 chopped banana.
Evening meal	1 portion *Chipotle Lentils* with 1 portion *Coconut Rice*, 1 (50g), 1 reduced-fat mini naan and 90g green beans or broccoli; 1 portion *Autumn Fruit Salad*.
Nutrition	**1788kcal, 54g fat and 7 portions of fruit and vegetables.**

Day 4

Breakfast	*Greek Yogurt with Berries and Walnuts*; 1 *Maple and Raisin Drop Scone* spread with 1 tsp (5g) olive spread.
Mid-morning	Glass of milk from allowance.
Midday meal	*Roasted Pepper and Halloumi Panini with Watercress and Clementine Salad*; 4 cherry tomatoes; 1 all-butter chocolate chip cookie (M&S).
Afternoon	200ml pressed apple juice.
Evening meal	1 portion *Mediterranean Fish in Filo Parcels* with 1 portion *Okra with Tomatoes*; 1 portion *Baked Plums with Port*; 125ml glass dry white wine.
Nutrition	**1789kcal, 56.6g fat and 6 to 7 portions of fruit and vegetables.**

Day 5

Breakfast	Half a grapefruit, 50g crunchy oat cereal with 1 tbsp added sunflower seeds and 150g low-fat plain yogurt.
Mid-morning	1 *Orange and Sour Cherry Muffin*.
Midday meal	*Piquant Egg and Watercress Sandwich* or retail equivalent with 365kcal and <11.5g fat; 25g bag baked crisps; 1 ripe mango, cubed.
Afternoon	1 large kiwi fruit.
Evening meal	1 portion *Home-made Burgers with Spicy Potato Wedges*; 1 tbsp *Spicy Harissa Dressing*; 6 cherry tomatoes and few slices cucumber; 1 *Passion Fruit Crème Caramel*.
Nutrition	**1810kcal, 53g fat and 5 portions of fruit and vegetables.**

Day 6

Breakfast	*Smoked Salmon with Baby Dill Pancakes*; 200ml orange juice; 125g summerfruit compote (bought) with 1 rounded tbsp (45g) Greek yogurt.
Mid-morning	80g grapes.
Midday meal	1 portion *Bacon and Sweetcorn Chowder* with 1 *Sundried Tomato and Black Olive Scone*.
Afternoon	1 sachet soup having 70kcal and <2g fat.
Evening meal	1 portion *Marinated Lamb with Crushed Potatoes*; 80g petits pois; 1 portion *Pear and Chocolate Pudding*.
Nutrition	**1800kcal, 52.3g fat and 6 portions of fruit and vegetables.**

Day 7

Breakfast	1 portion *Breakfast Compote*; 1 medium plain (60g) croissant.
Mid-morning	60g fromage frais.
Midday meal	1 portion *Chive Dip*; 1 portion *Home-made Houmous* with 2 soft breadsticks (Sainsbury's), 1 carrot cut into batons and half a sliced red pepper; 175ml glass dry red wine.
Afternoon	Glass of milk from allowance.
Evening meal	1 portion *Gammon with Sweet-and-sour Shallots* with 1 portion *Boulangère Potatoes*, 90g boiled sweetcorn and 85g steamed broccoli.
Nutrition	**1779kcal, 49.2g fat and 6 portions of fruit and vegetables.**

Also included: each day you may have 300ml skimmed milk (or non-dairy equivalent) for cereals and drinks. Drink at least 1.5 litres (6 x 250ml glasses) of water a day. Drinks such as juices, smoothies, alcohol etc. are not included unless stated.

Chapter 4

Recipes

This chapter provides you with nearly 200 tasty recipes, which are suitable for the time you are on the diet and beyond.

To help you find your way around the recipes they are split into the following sections:

- Breakfasts and Brunches
- Soups
- Sandwiches and Light Lunches
- Main course salads
- Poultry – chicken, turkey, duck
- Meat – beef, pork, lamb, venison
- Fish and seafood – white and oily fish, shellfish and other seafood
- Vegetarian
- Sides – those accompaniments for your meal, whether starchy, vegetables or salads
- Pasta
- Sauces, dressings and dips – to add extra zest to your meals
- Desserts
- Bites – scones, muffins and snacks

The recipes have been devised and kitchen-tested, and then nutritionally analysed by software designed specifically for this function. The diet allows you to follow a range of different calorie and fat bands, and the recipes reflect this, some being higher in calories and fat and others lower. On pages 286 to 292 you will find a list of all the recipes ordered by their fat content and another with their calorie content. This is to enable you to choose easily, not only by the type of recipe you fancy, but also by their nutritional value.

Some recipes provide one portion, while others provide for 2, 4 or (very occasionally) 6 portions. Many people who are on a diet are also the cook for their household, so the recipes have been written to make them as family-friendly as possible, with simple instructions and to minimize time in the kitchen. Storage instructions have also been provided, so if you make a dish that serves 4 but eat only one portion, you can save the remainder for another day.

Don't forget to weigh out or measure all the ingredients so that you meet your diet goals.

Hints for Lower-fat Cooking

There are lots of ways to cut down on fat in your diet, and tips are included here so you can use them when cooking. They fall broadly into three categories: the food you buy, how you cook it and the equipment you use to do so.

Ingredients

- Use reduced- or no-fat ingredients – semi- or skimmed milk, reduced-fat creams and yogurts. (See Chapter 9 for more information.)
- Spreads come in a range of different fat levels from 20–80 per cent fat. Use the lowest you can, remembering that if you cook with them, the lower the fat, the more water is present, so they may splutter if you try to fry with them.
- Oils are all almost 100 per cent fat. Choose unsaturated oils such as rapeseed and olive oil, which are high in monounsaturates, or polyunsaturated sunflower or corn oil. Most vegetable oil is rapeseed.
- If you are using cheese, use a reduced-fat version where you can. You can usually use less cheese if it tastes strong, so mature cheddar and parmesan will taste more evident in recipes than a mild cheddar or Edam.

- Choose the leanest meat you can afford, and trim off any visible fat. Cheaper lean cuts make great stews.
- Don't add oil to the pan when you are browning mince – let it brown in its own fat.
- When you are cooking chicken, if it has the skin on remove it before you cook if it is a stew or stir-fry, but if you are grilling keep it on to prevent the meat from drying out, then take it off before serving.
- Weigh and measure diligently. They may look innocent but flavourings such as pesto, sundried tomato paste, coconut milk or block coconut and curry paste all contain fat, so measure them out.

Cooking Methods

Lower-fat needn't mean zero fat, but it is important to control the amount of fat you use when cooking. Some cooking methods such as stewing and steaming rely on moisture rather than adding fat, and others use dry heat such as grilling and baking.

- When making a casserole or stew it is not always necessary to sear or brown the meat in oil first. Delicious stews can be made 'from cold', just placing all the ingredients in a casserole and popping it into the oven on a low heat to cook. You can use cheaper cuts of lean meat this way.
- Fish or poultry can be steamed in a foil parcel, which keeps the food moist and avoids adding fat.
- Fish and poultry can be gently poached in water, wine or milk. Adding herbs or citrus zest adds flavour. The poaching stock can then be thickened with cornflour for a sauce.
- Microwave ovens often have a range of settings, and microwaving can be a great way to cook fish as moisture is retained and the food is cooked quickly, helping to preserve vitamins.
- Grilling or barbecuing food uses high temperatures, so food that is naturally low in fat may need to be sprayed lightly with oil or marinated in low-fat ingredients to prevent it from drying out.
- Baking or roasting, like grilling, is great for many foods, but you may need to protect the food with foil, or lightly spray with oil.

- Stir-fried food can be higher in fat than you expect, so if you like to stir-fry, invest in a non-stick wok and measure out 1 tablespoon of oil to do the initial frying. If food starts to stick add water rather than more oil.
- Dry frying is useful for foods that contain some fat, to which you don't want to add any more. Bacon and mince are easily dry fried over a gentle heat in a non-stick pan.
- Griddling was traditionally used for cooking foods such as drop scones, but recently griddle pans or hob attachments have been designed with ridges so that fat can drain away from foods that contain fat. Oily fish like tuna or salmon, poultry, chops and steak as well as vegetables such as courgettes and peppers can be successfully griddled.

Equipment

There are several pieces of equipment that will make your life easier and add to your cooking experience. If you can, invest in these:

- Measuring spoons. 1 level teaspoon is very different from 1 heaped teaspoon when it is a high-fat ingredient, so buy a set of measuring spoons.
- Electronic scales. These will help you measure out ingredients accurately. Scales that can be reset to zero once a pan or bowl is on top are very useful.
- An oil spray or 'mister' that you can fill with rapeseed or olive oil will help you cut down on your usage of oil even more than measuring it out with a teaspoon.
- Non-stick pans. Buy yourself at least one heavy pan that is large enough to brown mince, or cook a stew.
- Sharp knives and a knife sharpener. Trimming off fat relies on a good knife, so either treat yourself to a new one, or buy a sharpener to improve the ones you already have.
- A hand blender/wand blender. If you don't have one of these gadgets already you will be surprised at how useful they are. Because you can put the blender in the pan, making soups becomes so much easier, and you can make shakes and knock lumps out of sauces and gravies quickly, too.

Breakfasts and Brunches

Breakfast Compote

Serves: 4   **Prep:** 5 minutes   **Cook:** Soak overnight
205kcal and 0.4g fat per portion

Start your day with a bowl of orange-soaked fruit. There is sufficient for 4 portions, so refrigerate any that remains, or have another portion as a dessert with your main meal.

100g dried or ready-
  to-eat apricots
100g raisins or
  sultanas
50g dried apple rings
50g dried sweetened
  cranberries
300ml unsweetened
  orange juice

1. **Place all the ingredients in a large bowl or jug and cover.**
2. **Leave in a cool place overnight.**
3. **Serve in the morning, and refrigerate any remaining.**

Serving Suggestions: Top with a rounded tbsp (35g) of low-fat plain yogurt: 225kcal and 0.7g fat

Storage: May be kept in an airtight container in the fridge for 2–3 days. Not suitable for freezing.

NUTRITIONAL ANALYSIS	Protein g	2.2	Fat g	0.4	Sodium g	Trace
PER PORTION	Carbohydrate g	50.9	Of which saturates g	0.0	Salt g	Trace
Energy kcal 205	Of which sugars g	49.7	Fibre g	6.0	Portion fruit and veg	1

Smoked Salmon with Baby Dill Pancakes

Serves: 4   **Prep:** 10 minutes   **Cook:** 10 minutes
290kcal and 10.8g fat per portion

A luxurious brunch recipe using a savoury pancake recipe. The baby pancakes are also delicious served with soup, and are great as a snack by themselves.

For 8 Pancakes

150g self-raising flour

150ml skimmed milk

1 medium egg

1 tbsp chopped fresh dill or 1 tsp dried

1 tbsp sunflower oil

For 1 Portion

2 pancakes

25g smoked salmon, cut into strips

30g extra-light soft cheese

25g cucumber slices

25g watercress

1. **Place the flour, milk, egg, dill and oil in a food processor and blend to mix to a batter.**
2. **Heat a griddle or flattish non-stick frying pan and spray lightly with oil.**
3. **Spoon the batter into the hot pan and gently cook until the top of the pancake is starting to dry. Turn over with a palette knife or non-stick spatula and cook for another minute or two. You should be able to make 8 pancakes.**
4. **Serve warm spread with the soft cheese, topped with the salmon and with the cucumber and watercress on the side.**

Serving Suggestions: Try the pancake alone with soup, or for a snack. 1 baby pancake has 95kcal and 2.8g fat.

Storage: The pancakes can be stored for a day or two in the fridge and also are suitable for freezing.

NUTRITIONAL ANALYSIS	Protein g		17.7	Fat g	10.8	Sodium g	0.3
PER PORTION	Carbohydrate g		32.6	Of which saturates g	2.6	Salt g	0.8
Energy kcal	290	Of which sugars g	4	Fibre g	2.0	Portion fruit and veg	½

Buttermilk Pancakes

Makes: 10 Pancakes   **Prep:** 5 minutes   **Cook:** 10 minutes
95kcal and 3g fat per portion

Delicious eaten hot from the griddle as a snack, for breakfast, or with compote as a dessert, these pancakes are sure to feature in your diet.

150g self-raising
 flour
284g carton
 buttermilk
1 egg, beaten
25g sugar
25g butter, melted
1 tsp grated lemon
 rind

1. Sieve the flour into a large jug or mixing bowl.
2. Stir in the buttermilk, beaten egg and sugar, and beat well.
3. Now add the melted butter and lemon rind to make a smooth, thick batter.
4. Heat a non-stick frying pan or flat griddle pan and spray lightly with cooking oil.
5. Using a tablespoon, drop the batter onto the hot pan. You will probably only get 3 or 4 in a pan at once.
6. Cook over a medium heat until the surface is drying and the bottom golden brown. Turn over and cook on the other side.
7. Continue with the remaining mixture until all are cooked.

Serving Suggestions: For breakfast try with a drizzle of maple syrup and a squirt of lime juice: 240kcal and 6g fat for 2.

For a dessert, top two with 1 tbsp (40g) Summer Fruit Compote (see page 255 for the recipe) and 1 tsp (10g) of reduced-fat crème fraîche. 240kcal and 8.0g fat.

Storage: The pancakes can be stored in the fridge in an airtight container for two days, or can be frozen. Separate with greaseproof paper or film to prevent sticking together.

NUTRITIONAL ANALYSIS	Protein g	3	Fat g	3	Sodium g	Trace
PER PANCAKE	Carbohydrate g	15.3	Of which saturates g	1.6	Salt g	Trace
Energy kcal 95	Of which sugars g	11.1	Fibre g	.6	Portion fruit and veg	0

Four-grain Porridge with Apricots

Serves: 2   **Prep:** 1 minute   **Cook:** 5 minutes

315kcal and 3.8g fat per portion

Delicious creamy-tasting porridge to start the day, which is low in GI so will keep any hunger pangs at bay. If you can't buy four-grain porridge, then use jumbo porridge oats. You can easily halve the recipe if it is just for you, but you may find all the family are keen to try this one, so you might need to double it!

60g dried apricots

100g four-grain porridge

200ml semi-skimmed milk

1. **Chop the apricots and place in a non-stick saucepan with the porridge oats and milk.**
2. **Slowly bring to the boil, stirring frequently and allowing the porridge to thicken – 4–5 minutes over a gentle heat.**
3. **Serve at once.**

Serving Suggestions: Serve as it is, or if you like add a little honey and milk.

Storage: Not suitable for storage.

As recipe

NUTRITIONAL ANALYSIS PER PORTION		Protein g	12	Fat g	3.8	Sodium g	Trace
		Carbohydrate g	62	Of which saturates g	2.2	Salt g	Trace
Energy kcal	315	Of which sugars g	28.9	Fibre g	2.7	Portion fruit and veg	1

With 50ml semi-skimmed milk and 1 tsp honey

NUTRITIONAL ANALYSIS PER PORTION		Protein g	10.3	Fat g	3	Sodium g	Trace
		Carbohydrate g	50.3	Of which saturates g	1.7	Salt g	Trace
Energy kcal	260	Of which sugars g	17.3	Fibre g	2.7	Portion fruit and veg	1

Grapefruit Salad with Toasted Almonds

Serves: 2   **Prep:** 10 minutes
220kcal and 11.5g fat per portion

Grapefruit is guaranteed to wake you up! If you can't face preparing it in the morning, do it the night before and store in the fridge, or use canned grapefruit segments in fruit juice.

1 red grapefruit
1 white or pink
  grapefruit or 320g
  can grapefruit in
  fruit juice, drained
32g (4 level tsp) runny
  honey
40g toasted almonds

1. **Peel the grapefruit using a sharp knife, and then, holding the fruit over a bowl to catch any juice, carefully cut the grapefruit into segments, discarding the inner membranes.**
2. **Drizzle the honey over the grapefruit and sprinkle over the toasted almonds.**
3. **Serve at once.**

Serving Suggestions: Top with a rounded tbsp of fat-free Greek yogurt: 245kcal and 11.5g fat.

Storage: You can store the fruit in the fridge for 24 hours without the almonds, but it will lose some vitamin C.

NUTRITIONAL ANALYSIS		Protein g	5.6	Fat g	11.5	Sodium g	Trace
PER PORTION		Carbohydrate g	24.5	Of which saturates g	0.9	Salt g	Trace
Energy kcal	220	Of which sugars g	24	Fibre g	3.6	Portion fruit and veg	1

Greek Yogurt with Berries and Walnuts

Serves: 1   **Prep:** 5 minutes

295kcal and 13.9g fat per portion

Fat-free Greek yogurt keeps the saturates as well as the fat down, so you can have healthier unsaturated fat from the nuts. If you use a teaspoon that you have just dipped into boiling water, you will be able to measure the honey fairly easily.

100g mixed berries, 1 or more of strawberries, raspberries, blueberries, blackberries

150g pot fat-free Greek yogurt

20g walnuts, chopped

20g (2 tsp) runny honey

1. **Prepare the berries by washing and hulling if necessary.**
2. **Place the yogurt in a bowl, and sprinkle over the berries.**
3. **Add the chopped nuts, and lastly drizzle over the honey.**
4. **Serve at once.**

Serving Suggestions: Serve with a glass of fruit juice.

Nutrition without the walnuts: 160kcal and 0.3g fat.

Storage: Not suitable for storage.

NUTRITIONAL ANALYSIS		Protein g	17.4	Fat g	13.9	Sodium g	trace
PER PORTION		Carbohydrate g	26.9	Of which saturates g	1.3	Salt g	Trace
Energy kcal	295	Of which sugars g	26.7	Fibre g	4.0	Portion fruit and veg	1

Ham and Cheese Toastie

Serves: 1   **Prep:** 5 minutes   **Cook:** 3–4 minutes

380kcal and 11.6g fat per portion

You don't need lots of butter to make a toastie, especially if you have a sandwich toaster. Using reduced-fat cheese means you can have a larger portion of it, for additional calcium without extra fat.

72g (2 medium slices) granary bread

15g (1 level tbsp) tomato relish

35g slice of premium ham

50g reduced-fat cheddar, sliced

90g (about 6) cherry tomatoes

1. Spread 1 slice of the bread with the relish and top with the ham.
2. Place the sliced cheese on top of the ham and add the second piece of bread.
3. Place in a sandwich toaster and cook until browned, or gently cook in a non-stick frying pan, spraying with a little oil.
4. Serve with the tomatoes.

Serving Suggestions: Try with a bowl of soup for a delicious lunch.

Storage: Not suitable for storage.

NUTRITIONAL ANALYSIS		Protein g	31	Fat g	11.6	Sodium g	1.2
PER PORTION		Carbohydrate g	37.5	Of which saturates g	6.1	Salt g	3
Energy kcal	380	Of which sugars g	8.4	Fibre g	2.6	Portion fruit and veg	1

Poached Egg Muffin
with Spinach and Mushrooms

Serves: 1   **Prep:** 5 minutes   **Cook:** 15 minutes

300kcal and 12.8g fat per portion

At the weekend, why not make yourself brunch with this tasty egg muffin? Add a glass of juice or a smoothie to complete the meal.

1 tsp olive oil

50g mushrooms, sliced

50g baby spinach leaves

1 medium egg

1 English muffin

1 tsp (5g) low-fat (<40% fat) spread

Black pepper and nutmeg to season

1. Heat the oil in a non-stick pan and very gently cook the mushrooms until soft, about 8–10 minutes.

2. Add the spinach, cover and allow it to wilt, then season and remove from the heat.

3. Meanwhile, poach the egg.

4. Halve and toast the muffin and spread one side with the spread.

5. Using a slotted serving spoon, lift the spinach and mushroom from the pan, allowing any cooking liquid to drain off, and place on the 'unbuttered' muffin half.

6. Top with the poached egg and use the other muffin half to make a lid.

7. Serve at once.

Serving Suggestions: Served with a 200ml glass of unsweetened orange juice: 370kcal and 12.9g fat.

Storage: Not suitable for storage.

NUTRITIONAL ANALYSIS PER PORTION		Protein g	18.2	Fat g	12.8	Sodium g	0.5
		Carbohydrate g	28.2	Of which saturates g	3	Salt g	1.3
Energy kcal	300	Of which sugars g	3.1	Fibre g	2.9	Portion fruit and veg	1

Scrambled Egg on Toast

Serves: 1 **Prep:** 5 minutes **Cook:** 10 minutes
310kcal and 11.7g fat per portion

For those mornings when you have a little time, why not enjoy a cooked breakfast? Using spread that contains 40g fat per 100g (40% fat) helps keep this within your fat targets.

80g baby plum
  tomatoes, halved
1 medium egg
25ml skimmed milk
Black pepper
10g (2 tsp) 40% fat
  polyunsaturated
  spread
72g (2 medium slices)
  granary bread,
  toasted

1. **Place the tomatoes under a preheated grill.**
2. **Beat the egg and milk with pepper, and melt 1 teaspoon of the spread in a non-stick pan.**
3. **Gently cook the scrambled egg, stirring often until it set.**
4. **Place on top of a piece of 'unbuttered' toast. Use the remaining spread on the other piece of toast.**
5. **Serve with the grilled tomatoes.**

Serving Suggestions: Add a glass of fruit juice or a bowl of chopped fresh fruit to complete your breakfast.

Storage: Not suitable for storage.

NUTRITIONAL ANALYSIS		Protein g	15.6	Fat g	11.7	Sodium g	0.5
PER PORTION		Carbohydrate g	38	Of which saturates g	3	Salt g	1.25
Energy kcal	310	Of which sugars g	5.9	Fibre g	5.6	Portion fruit and veg	1

Breakfast Smoothie

Serves: 1   **Prep:** 5 minutes

160kcal and 1.8g fat per portion

Wake up to this delicious smoothie, which will slip down easily, providing you with calcium, B vitamins and vitamin C in a few tasty gulps.

150g low-fat (<3% fat) plain yogurt

2 passion fruit, seeds scooped into a sieve and juice pressed through

55ml juice of one small freshly squeezed orange

50g (half) a medium banana

1. **Place all the ingredients in a blender or food processor and blend until smooth.**

2. **Serve at once.**

Serving Suggestions: Drink straight away to help you wake up!

Storage: Can be stored for 24 hours in the fridge, though may separate.

NUTRITIONAL ANALYSIS		Protein g	8.9	Fat g	1.8	Sodium g	0.1
PER PORTION		Carbohydrate g	28.9	Of which saturates g	1.1	Salt g	0.2
Energy kcal	160	Of which sugars g	27.3	Fibre g	2.0	Portion fruit and veg	1

Soups

Bacon and Sweetcorn Chowder

Serves: 2 **Prep:** 5 minutes **Cook:** 30 minutes

320kcal and 13g fat per portion

This really is a meal in itself rather than a soup to preface a meal. It is colourful, tasty and easy, so enjoy!

100g lean back bacon, trimmed of fat and diced

30g (1 large or 2 small) spring onions, chopped

250g potatoes, peeled and diced

150g frozen sweetcorn

300ml water

2 bay leaves

40g (1 rounded tbsp) reduced-fat crème fraîche

1 tsp chopped fresh parsley

Black pepper

1. Heat the bacon in a non-stick saucepan to allow it to brown.
2. After 3–4 minutes add the spring onions and potatoes.
3. Stir in the sweetcorn, water and bay leaves, and bring to the boil.
4. Simmer for 20 minutes or until the potatoes are soft and have started to thicken the chowder.
5. Remove from the heat, and stir in the crème fraîche, parsley and black pepper to taste.
6. Serve at once.

Serving Suggestions: Add a bread roll to complete your meal.

Storage: Not suitable for freezing, but can be stored for up to 2 days in the fridge.

NUTRITIONAL ANALYSIS PER PORTION		Protein g	15.2	Fat g	13	Sodium g	0.5
		Carbohydrate g	37	Of which saturates g	5.3	Salt g	0.1
Energy kcal	320	Of which sugars g	3.2	Fibre g	4.0	Portion fruit and veg	1

Watercress Soup

Serves: 3   **Prep:** 10 minutes   **Cook:** 20 minutes

110kcal and 4.7g fat per portion

Watercress is an excellent source of beta-carotene, vitamin C and also provides folate. It doesn't really need to be cooked in this soup, just wilted, which also preserves some of the vitamins.

1 tbsp olive oil

140g (1 medium) leek, finely sliced

200g (1 medium) potato, diced

600ml water

1 tsp reduced-sodium vegetable bouillon

150g watercress, washed and large stalks removed

Black pepper

1. In a large non-stick saucepan heat the oil and sweat the leek for 5 minutes.
2. Add the potato, water and bouillon, and bring to the boil, stirring occasionally.
3. Cover, reduce the heat and simmer for 20 minutes or until the potatoes are tender.
4. Stir in the watercress and remove from the heat to allow the cress to wilt. Season.
5. Blend until smooth.
6. Serve at once.

Serving Suggestions: Serve with a crusty roll and soft cheese.

Storage: Can be stored in the fridge in an airtight container for 2 days. Reheat until piping hot. Can also be frozen.

NUTRITIONAL ANALYSIS		Protein g	3.8	Fat g	4.7	Sodium g	0.1
PER PORTION		Carbohydrate g	13.6	Of which saturates g	0.7	Salt g	0.25
Energy kcal	110	Of which sugars g	2	Fibre g	2.6	Portion fruit and veg	1

Cauliflower and Almond Soup

Serves: 6 **Prep:** 5 minutes **Cook:** 25 minutes

125kcal and 4.5g fat per portion

A mild and creamy soup that is scented with bay leaves. It is a great source of calcium from both the milk and the almonds.

500ml skimmed milk

10g (2 tsp) reduced-salt vegetable bouillon

500ml water

160g (1 medium) onion, roughly chopped

4 bay leaves

1kg cauliflower florets, roughly chopped

30g ground almonds

Freshly grated nutmeg to taste

1. Place the milk, bouillon powder and water in a large saucepan.
2. Add the onion, bay leaves and cauliflower.
3. Bring slowly to the boil, cover and allow to simmer for 20 minutes.
4. When the vegetables are soft, remove from the heat and blend until smooth.
5. Return to the pan and add the ground almonds. Add nutmeg to taste.
6. Stir through and serve.

Serving Suggestions: This soup is very pale in colour, so serve in brightly coloured soup bowls with croutons made by drying bread cubes in the oven.

Storage: This soup can be refrigerated for up to 2 days in an airtight container. It also freezes well.

NUTRITIONAL ANALYSIS	Protein g	10.2	Fat g	4.5	Sodium g	<0.1
PER PORTION	Carbohydrate g	11.1	Of which saturates g	0.6	Salt g	0.2
Energy kcal	125	Of which sugars g	9.5	Fibre g	3.7	Portion fruit and veg	1

Chinese-style Soup with Tiny Pork Balls

Serves: 4 starters   **Prep:** 10 minutes   **Cook:** 15 minutes
112kcal and 3.2g fat per portion

A simple soup that uses the Pork Patties recipe (on page 161) for the tiny balls, so one mixture covers two meals. This is a starter-size portion, but if you are hungry why not make it a main meal by doubling the mixture and adding a bread roll?

750g good-quality chicken stock.

30g celery (1 stick), finely sliced

80g red pepper (about half), finely sliced

30g (about 3) spring onions, chopped into 1-cm slices

60g fine rice noodles

1 tbsp fish sauce

¼ of the Pork Patties mixture (134g) – see page 161 for recipe

Black pepper

250ml water

1. **Place the stock in a large saucepan or wok and bring to the boil.**

2. **Add the celery, pepper and spring onions, and simmer for 5 minutes.**

3. **Add the rice noodles and fish sauce, and continue to cook for 2–3 minutes.**

4. **Meanwhile divide the Pork Patties mixture into 8 small balls and drop into the hot soup.**

5. **Boil gently for 5 minutes until the pork balls are cooked through. Season.**

6. **Serve at once.**

Storage: Best served straight away to retain vitamin content of soup, but can be stored for 1 day in the fridge. Must be reheated until piping hot.

NUTRITIONAL ANALYSIS		Protein g	6.5	Fat g	3.2	Sodium mg	0.8
PER PORTION		Carbohydrate g	14.3	Of which saturates g	1.1	Salt g	2
Energy kcal	112	Of which sugars g	1.7	Fibre g	0.8	Portion fruit and veg	0

Creamy Cherry Tomato Soup

Serves: 4   **Prep:** 5–10 minutes   **Cook:** 25 minutes

111kcal and 6.3g fat per serving

This soup is a lovely standby to keep in the freezer or fridge. You can make a lower-fat version by leaving out the crème fraîche. Serve it with cubes of bread crisped up in the oven.

1 tsp olive oil

1 medium (160g) onion, finely chopped

2 sticks (75g) celery

750g ripe cherry tomatoes

35g (1 rounded tbsp) tomato purée

1 tsp sugar

350ml chicken or vegetable stock

400ml water

Black pepper

100g reduced-fat crème fraîche

1. Heat the oil in a large non-stick saucepan and gently sweat the onion and celery, stirring frequently for 5 minutes.
2. Wash the cherry tomatoes and tip into the pan along with the tomato purée and sugar.
3. Add the stock and water. (If you are using a stock cube, just use half and 750ml of water to keep the salt level down.)
4. Bring to the boil and then cover, and reduce the heat. Simmer for 20 minutes, stirring occasionally to burst the tomatoes.
5. Blend until smooth. If you like very smooth soup, press it through a fairly coarse sieve.
6. Off the heat, stir in the crème fraîche and serve at once.

Serving Suggestions: Serve with bread rolls spread with low-fat soft cheese and crunchy celery.

Storage: Can be refrigerated for 2–3 days or frozen.

With crème fraîche

NUTRITIONAL ANALYSIS PER PORTION		Protein g	3.1	Fat g	6.3	Sodium mg	240
		Carbohydrate g	11.4	Of which saturates g	3.3	Salt g	0.6
Kcal	111	Of which sugars g	10.5	Fibre g	2.7	Portion fruit and veg	1½

Without crème fraîche

NUTRITIONAL ANALYSIS PER PORTION		Protein g	2.3	Fat g	1.8	Sodium mg	240
		Carbohydrate g	10.7	Of which saturates g	0.3	Salt g	0.6
Kcal	68	Of which sugars g	9.8	Fibre g	2.7	Portion fruit and veg	1½

Curried Parsnip and Apple Soup

Serves: 4   **Prep:** 5 minutes with a processor   **Cook:** 25 minutes
140kcal and 5.4g fat per portion

A great soup to have in the freezer for cold days when you need warming up.

160g (1 medium) onion, peeled and quartered

1 tbsp rapeseed oil

450g parsnips, peeled

10g (1 heaped tsp) curry paste

750ml water

200g (1 medium) cooking apple, peeled and cored

1. If you are using a food processor, place the onion in the bowl and chop until fine. Alternatively chop finely with a knife.

2. Heat the oil in a large non-stick saucepan and soften the onion for a few minutes.

3. Meanwhile chop the parsnips in the processor until fine, or grate.

4. Add the parsnips to the pan and stir in the curry paste and water.

5. Lastly chop the apple and add to the mixture.

6. Bring to the boil, cover and simmer for 25 minutes until the vegetables are tender.

7. Blend to make a smooth, thick soup, adding a little boiling water if it is too thick.

Serving Suggestions: Serve with a few dried apple crisps on top and a crusty roll.

Storage: Can be frozen and also will keep in the fridge for 2–3 days in an airtight container.

NUTRITIONAL ANALYSIS		Protein g	2.7	Fat g	5.4	Sodium g	<0.1
PER PORTION		Carbohydrate g	20.8	Of which saturates g	0.7	Salt g	0.1
Energy kcal	140	Of which sugars g	12.1	Fibre g	7.1	Portion fruit and veg	1

Moroccan Chickpea and Fruit Soup

Serves: 4   **Prep:** 15 minutes   **Cook:** 30 minutes

185kcal and 4.3g fat per portion

A host of flavours combine to make this soup taste really special. It is almost a meal in itself, just needing some crusty bread to accompany it.

1 tbsp olive oil

320g (2 medium) onions, finely chopped

3 cloves garlic, crushed

1 tsp ground cinnamon

½ tsp chilli powder

2 tsp ground cumin

400g can chickpeas in water, drained

150g dried apricots, roughly chopped

Grated zest of 1 orange

150ml orange juice

Juice of 1 lemon

75g frozen chopped spinach, defrosted

1 tsp reduced-salt vegetable bouillon

600ml water

1. **Heat the oil and fry the onions and garlic in a large non-stick pan for 5 minutes until softened.**
2. **Add the spices and fry for another minute or two, adding a little water if they start to stick.**
3. **Stir in all the remaining ingredients and bring to the boil, stirring occasionally.**
4. **Simmer, covered, for 20–25 minutes, stirring occasionally.**
5. **You may want to leave this soup chunky or blend a little for a thickly textured soup. If it is too thick, dilute with a little boiling water.**
6. **Serve at once.**

Serving Suggestions: Leave the lemon juice out of the recipe and pour over the soup as you serve.

Storage: Can be frozen and refrigerated for up to 3 days. Don't forget that vitamin C declines on storage, so if you are not going to eat it within 24 hours, freezing may be a better option.

NUTRITIONAL ANALYSIS	Protein g	8.2	Fat g	4.3	Sodium g	0.1
PER PORTION	Carbohydrate g	30.3	Of which saturates g	0.5	Salt g	0.2
Energy kcal 185	Of which sugars g	20.6	Fibre g	7.4	Portion fruit and veg	2½

Pea Soup with Pesto Croute

Serves: 4   **Prep:** 10 minutes   **Cook:** 15 minutes
170kcal and 5.5g fat per portion

A very easy soup to make, which is also rich in vitamin C, served with a single pesto-covered croute.

2 tsp rapeseed oil

80g (8) spring onions, roughly chopped

450g petits pois, defrosted

600ml water

2 tsp reduced-sodium vegetable bouillon

Few mint leaves

For the croutes

100g baguette, sliced into 4 pieces

20g (4 level tsp) pesto

1. **Preheat oven to 200°C/180°C Fan/GM5.**
2. **Heat the oil in a non-stick pan and gently fry the spring onions.**
3. **After a few minutes add the peas, water and stock, and bring to the boil.**
4. **Add the mint leaves, cover and reduce the heat.**
5. **Simmer the soup for 10 minutes, then remove from the heat and blend until smooth.**
6. **Meanwhile place the bread in a hot oven to become crisp – about 10 minutes – and spread each slice with 1 teaspoon of pesto.**
7. **Serve the soup with a pesto croute floating in the centre of each bowl.**

Serving Suggestions: Without the pesto croutes the soup provides 75kcal and 2.6g fat per portion.

Storage: The soup can be stored for 2 days in the fridge in an airtight container and can also be frozen.

NUTRITIONAL ANALYSIS		Protein g	8.8	Fat g	5.5	Sodium g	0.2
PER PORTION		Carbohydrate g	22.1	Of which saturates g	0.7	Salt g	0.5
Energy kcal	170	Of which sugars g	4.7	Fibre g	5.3	Portion fruit and veg	1

Pumpkin Soup

Serves: 4   **Prep:** 15 minutes   **Cook:** 20 minutes
105kcal and 4.9g fat per portion

Pumpkin is a great source of beta-carotene – the plant form of vitamin A that helps protect body cells against damage. If you can't buy fresh pumpkin or don't have time to prepare it, look for cans of ready-prepared pumpkin purée.

Ingredients	Method
2 tsp olive oil	1. Heat the oil in a large non-stick saucepan and gently fry the onion for a few minutes.
160g (1 medium) onion, finely chopped	
1 tsp ground ginger	2. Stir in the spices and pumpkin, and then add the stock.
1 tsp ground cumin	3. Bring the mixture to the boil, then cover and simmer for 15–20 minutes until the pumpkin is tender.
1 tsp grated nutmeg	
1kg peeled and seeded pumpkin, cut into cubes	
500ml vegetable stock	4. Blend the soup until smooth then add the grated nutmeg.
50g half-fat crème fraîche	5. Stir in the crème fraîche just before serving.

Serving Suggestions: Serve with a granary roll filled with low-fat soft cheese and cucumber for a delicious lunch.

Storage: The soup will keep in the fridge for 2–3 days in an airtight container. It is also suitable for freezing.

NUTRITIONAL ANALYSIS PER PORTION						
Protein g	3	Fat g	4.9	Sodium g	0.3
Carbohydrate g	12.1	Of which saturates g	2.2	Salt g	0.75
Energy kcal	105	Of which sugars g	9.1	Fibre g	3.1	Portion fruit and veg	1

Carrot and Celery Soup

Serves: 4 **Prep:** 10 minutes **Cook:** 20 minutes
70kcal and 1.4g fat per portion

This is a very low-fat soup, which makes an excellent filler between meals when you are feeling peckish. If you have a food processor this soup is made even quicker if you chop or grate all the ingredients first.

1 tsp rapeseed oil
160g (1 medium) onion, finely chopped
60g celery, sliced
500g carrots, grated
700ml water
1 tsp reduced-sodium vegetable bouillon
Grated nutmeg
Few celery leaves (optional)

1. **Heat the oil in a large non-stick pan and gently fry the onion and celery for 5 minutes, stirring frequently.**
2. **Add the carrots, water and bouillon, and bring to the boil.**
3. **Cover and simmer for 20 minutes, stirring occasionally until all the vegetables are tender.**
4. **Either serve as is or, if you prefer a smooth soup, blend.**
5. **Grate a little nutmeg on top of each bowl, and sprinkle over some chopped celery leaves.**

Serving Suggestions: Make some croutons by drying some bread cubes in the oven and add a few to the soup.

Storage: Can be stored in the fridge in an airtight container for up to 3 days. Suitable for freezing.

NUTRITIONAL ANALYSIS		Protein g	1.7	Fat g	1.4	Sodium g	<0.1
PER PORTION		Carbohydrate g	13	Of which saturates g	0.2	Salt g	0.2
Energy kcal	70	Of which sugars g	11.5	Fibre g	4.0	Portion fruit and veg	1

Sandwiches and Light Lunches

Bacon- and Sweetcorn-stuffed Sweet Potato

Serves: 1 **Prep:** 10 minutes **Cook:** 60 minutes

335 kcal and 14.6g fat per portion

This has Saturday lunchtime written all over it! Sweet potatoes are a great source of vitamin A and are low in GI. Grilling the bacon keeps down the fat too.

130g sweet potato

50g (2 rashers) lean
  back bacon

60g sweetcorn,
  canned

15g sundried
  tomatoes in oil

35g (1 rounded tbsp)
  half-fat sour
  cream

40g rocket leaves

1. Bake the sweet potato in a hot oven (200°C/180°C Fan/GM 6) or microwave oven until soft.

2. Grill the bacon until crispy then chop.

3. Drain the sundried tomato and chop roughly. Mix it with the sweetcorn and cream, and then add the bacon.

4. Split open the potato, and add the bacon filling.

5. Serve with the rocket.

Serving suggestions: Use peas instead of sweetcorn.

Storage: The filling can be refrigerated for 24 hours.

NUTRITIONAL ANALYSIS PER PORTION:		Protein g	13.1	Fat g	14.6	Sodium g	1.3
		Carbohydrate g	37.6	Of which saturates g	4.7	Salt g	3.25
Energy kcal	335	Of which sugars g	19.7	Fibre g	5.4	Portion fruit and veg	1

Warm Wrap with Refried Beans, Avocado and Peppers

Serves: 2   **Prep:** 5 minutes   **Cook:** 5 minutes

380kcal and 13.8g fat per portion

This makes a lovely vegetarian lunch for two. Buy a baby avocado to make this so you won't be tempted to eat the leftovers from a large one. Avocado is a great source of essential vitamin E, but contains nearly 20g fat per 100g – hence sharing it!

215g can refried beans, e.g. Discovery

100g avocado (1 baby)

Juice of half a lemon

112g (2) multiseed tortilla wraps

80g (half) a red pepper, finely sliced

80g (half) a green pepper, finely sliced

30g rocket leaves

1. **Warm the beans, stirring all the time.**
2. **Cut the avocado into cubes and sprinkle with lemon juice.**
3. **Meanwhile warm or toast the wraps, then spread each with half the beans.**
4. **Add the peppers, avocado and rocket leaves.**
5. **Roll up each wrap and serve at once.**

Serving Suggestions: Omit the avocado and add 2 rounded tbsp reduced-fat sour cream per portion: 339kcal and 7.1g fat.

Storage: Not suitable for storage.

NUTRITIONAL ANALYSIS		Protein g	12.8	Fat g	13.8	Sodium g	0.7
PER PORTION		Carbohydrate g	57.6	Of which saturates g	3.8	Salt g	1.75
Energy kcal	390	Of which sugars g	8	Fibre g	9.6	Portion fruit and veg	2½

Baked Potato with Ratatouille and Goats Cheese

Serves: 1   **Prep:** 10 minutes   **Cook:** 60 minutes

430kcal and 10.9g fat per portion

This lunch uses the ratatouille recipe on page 221, though you can buy ratatouille if you prefer, checking the fat content as it may be higher than home made.

180g (1 medium) baking potato

350g ratatouille – either bought or ¼ recipe on page 221

50g goats cheese, e.g. Chavrou

1. Bake the potato in a hot oven (200°C/180°C Fan/GM6) or microwave oven until tender.
2. Meanwhile heat the ratatouille until piping hot.
3. Split the potato in half and mash the inside slightly with a fork. Spoon over the ratatouille.
4. Crumble the cheese on top and serve at once.

Serving Suggestions: If you don't like goats cheese, use feta or reduced-fat cheddar instead.

Storage: Not suitable for storage.

NUTRITIONAL ANALYSIS PER PORTION			Protein g	15.9	Fat g	10.9	Sodium g	0.2
			Carbohydrate g	75.5	Of which saturates g	6.5	Salt g	0.5
Energy kcal		430	Of which sugars g	17.2	Fibre g	7.8	Portion fruit and veg	3

Bruschetta with Mozzarella, Basil and Tomatoes

Serves: 2   **Prep:** 5 minutes   **Cook:** 5 minutes

310kcal and 10.8g fat per portion

Lovely for summer days when tomatoes are sweet and cheap, this lunch dish also provides you with over a third of your daily vitamin-C requirement. You can now buy reduced-fat mozzarella, so choose this over full fat.

130g (1 small baguette), halved lengthwise

1 clove garlic

2 tsp olive oil

160g ripe cherry tomatoes, halved or 2 medium tomatoes, skinned and chopped

125g light mozzarella (e.g. Sainsbury's BGTY), sliced thinly

5–6 basil leaves

Black pepper to taste

1. **Place the cut baguette in a hot oven (200°C/180°C Fan/ GM6) for 5–10 minutes to become really crispy.**
2. **Remove from the heat and rub with garlic, using the whole clove.**
3. **Drizzle over the olive oil and top with the tomatoes, mozzarella and torn basil leaves.**
4. **Grind a little pepper over and serve at once.**

Serving Suggestions: Serve with some fruit or a smoothie for a super-healthy lunch.

Storage: Not suitable for storage.

NUTRITIONAL ANALYSIS PER PORTION		Protein g	12.7	Fat g	10.8	Sodium g	0.4
		Carbohydrate g	39.6	Of which saturates g	5.3	Salt g	1
Energy kcal	310	Of which sugars g	5.1	Fibre g	0.1	Portion fruit and veg	1

Chicken Tikka Pitta with Raita

Serves: 1 **Prep:** 5 minutes

235kcal and 3.6g fat per portion

Spicy meat along with cooling raita, this delicious lunch is simple and low in fat. If you are buying raita you will need to check the fat and calorie content, but making it is very easy (see page 247).

60g (1) wholemeal pitta

60g (¼ recipe) home-made Raita (see page 247)

65g tikka roast chicken (from the deli section of your supermarket)

20g lettuce (or salad leaves of your choice)

1. **Warm the pitta and slice open.**
2. **Spread with the raita and pop in the chicken.**
3. **Add the lettuce and serve at once.**

Serving Suggestions: Add some fruit and a small bag of low-fat crisps or pretzels.

Storage: Not suitable for storage.

NUTRITIONAL ANALYSIS PER PORTION		Protein g	25.8	Fat g	3.6	Sodium g	0.4
		Carbohydrate g	24.5	Of which saturates g	0.8	Salt g	1
Energy kcal	235	Of which sugars g	3.6	Fibre g	0.4	Portion fruit and veg	1

Ciabatta Roll with Pesto, Soft Cheese and Baby Spinach

Serves: 1   **Prep:** 5 minutes

310kcal and 12.2g fat per portion

Pesto is strong in flavour so a little goes a long way. Measure it out to control your fat intake.

70g (1) ciabatta roll

30g extra light soft cheese (4% fat)

15g (1 level tbsp) pesto

15g (handful) baby spinach leaves

90g (6) cherry tomatoes

1. Cut the roll in half and spread both halves with the soft cheese, then add the pesto to one half.
2. Add the spinach leaves and replace the top.
3. Serve with the cherry tomatoes.

Serving Suggestions: Served with a 200ml glass of unsweetened fruit juice and 2 plums (100g): 430kcal and 12.6g fat.

Storage: Not suitable for storage.

NUTRITIONAL ANALYSIS		Protein g	11.8	Fat g	12.2	Sodium g	0.6
PER PORTION		Carbohydrate g	36.6	Of which saturates g	2.1	Salt g	1.5
Energy kcal	310	Of which sugars g	5.3	Fibre g	1.2	Portion fruit and veg	1

Ham and Caramelized Red Onion Chutney Sandwich

Serves: 1   **Prep:** 5 minutes

390kcal and 7.6g fat per portion

Lots of filling in good bread makes a really decent sandwich. This one won't disappoint.

72g (2 slices) wholemeal bread

10g (2 tsp) low-fat spread (40% fat)

50g (1 heaped tbsp) caramelized red onion chutney

60g (2 slices) good-quality ham

30g (half an average) beetroot (raw), peeled and grated, or 1 tomato, sliced

30g (1 small) stick celery

1. Spread the bread with the low-fat spread, then one side with the chutney.
2. Add the ham and grated beetroot or tomato then pop on the 'lid'.
3. Cut in half and serve at once with celery sticks.

Serving Suggestions: A ½ pint of lager would be a great accompaniment, but don't forget to add the calories (about 90kcal).

Storage: Not suitable for storage.

NUTRITIONAL ANALYSIS PER PORTION		Protein g	24.1	Fat g	7.6	Sodium g	1.1
		Carbohydrate g	56.1	Of which saturates g	9.6	Salt g	2.8
Energy kcal	390	Of which sugars g	26.6	Fibre g	5	Portion fruit and veg	1

Hot Prawn Tortilla Wrap

Serves: 1   **Prep:** 5 minutes   **Cook:** 2 minutes
305kcal and 7.1g fat per portion

This makes a delicious quick lunch or light supper.

1 soft flour tortilla
wrap (about 64g)

20g extra-light soft
cheese

1 tsp olive oil

1 clove garlic

40g cooked peeled
king prawns

Few sprigs of
watercress

1 apple, sliced

1. **Spread the tortilla with the soft cheese.**
2. **Heat the oil in a non-stick pan and stir-fry the garlic and prawns until hot – 2 minutes.**
3. **Place the prawns in the wrap and top with the watercress.**
4. **Fold the wrap and serve at once with slices of apple.**

Serving Suggestions: Complete your lunch with a low-fat yogurt and glass of fruit juice or a smoothie.

Storage: Not suitable for storing.

NUTRITIONAL ANALYSIS						
PER PORTION	Protein g	16.4	Fat g	7.1	Sodium mg	0.5
	Carbohydrate g	44.3	Of which saturates g	2	Salt g	1.1
Energy kcal	305	Of which sugars g	13.8	Fibre g	3.1	Portion fruit and veg	1

Mozzarella and Ham Panini

Serves: 1   **Prep:** 5 minutes   **Cook:** 5 minutes

315kcal and 15.6g fat per portion

A simple hot panini that can be made in a sandwich toaster or frying pan.

75g ciabatta

5g (1 level tsp) sundried tomato paste

20g slice of lean ham

20g grated mozzarella

2–3 basil leaves, torn

5–6 baby plum tomatoes

30g baby leaf salad

1. **Slice the ciabatta in half lengthwise and spread with the tomato paste.**
2. **Place the ham and grated mozzarella on the ciabatta, and top with the basil.**
3. **Place in a sandwich toaster for 4–5 minutes until the ciabatta is golden brown and the mozzarella melted.**
4. **Serve with the tomatoes and salad leaves.**

Serving Suggestions: Drizzle a little balsamic glaze or fat-free dressing over the salad. (Balsamic glaze is available in most supermarkets in the vinegars section – it is fat-free and is sure to become one of your cupboard staples once you've tried it.)

Storage: Not suitable for storage.

NUTRITIONAL ANALYSIS PER PORTION		Protein g	11.9	Fat g	15.6	Sodium mg	700
		Carbohydrate g	31.7	Of which saturates g	4.5	Salt g	1.8
Energy kcal	315	Of which sugars g	4.3	Fibre g	3.0	Portion fruit and veg	1

Piquant Egg and Watercress Sandwich

Serves: 1   **Prep:** 5 minutes   **Cook:** 10 minutes

365kcal and 11.3g fat per portion

A creamy egg filling with a bite from spring onions and peppadew peppers. Look for reduced-fat mayonnaise and mix it with fat-free Greek yogurt.

60g (1 large) egg

15g (1 level tbsp) reduced-fat mayonnaise

45g (1 rounded tbsp) fat-free Greek yogurt

30g (2–3) peppadew peppers, finely chopped

1 spring onion, chopped

80g (2 slices) half-white, half-wholemeal bread

20g watercress

1. **Hard boil the egg, then allow to cool in cold water.**
2. **Mix the mayonnaise with the yogurt, peppers and onion, and when the egg is cool peel and chop this into the mixture.**
3. **Spread the mixture on the bread, and add the watercress. Sandwich together, cut in half and serve.**

Serving Suggestions: Serve with a chopped apple or celery and carrot sticks.

Storage: May be stored in the fridge for 24 hours in an airtight container.

NUTRITIONAL ANALYSIS PER PORTION		Protein g	19.5	Fat g	11.3	Sodium g	0.9
		Carbohydrate g	48.6	Of which saturates g	2.5	Salt g	2.3
Energy kcal	365	Of which sugars g	14.5	Fibre g	4.4	Portion fruit and veg	½

Roasted Pepper and Halloumi Panini with Watercress and Clementine Salad

Serves: 1   **Prep:** 5 minutes   **Cook:** 5 minutes

414kcal and 13.2g fat per portion

Roasted vegetables in oil have always been popular antipasto, and some are available in balsamic vinegar instead. This one uses peppers in balsamic from Sainsbury's, but you could use grilled vegetables or semi-dried tomatoes in oil instead, looking out for varieties that contain less than 4g fat per 100g when drained.

20g watercress

1 large clementine or satuma, peeled and separated into segments

1 tbsp balsamic glaze

85g (1) panini roll

50g (drained weight) roasted pepper antipasto in balsamic vinegar

60g light halloumi cheese, sliced

1. **Make the salad by washing and drying the watercress, and removing any thick stalks.**
2. **On a serving plate mix together the watercress and clementine or satsuma, and drizzle over the balsamic.**
3. **Cut the panini in half and fill with the roasted pepper and halloumi, then place in a sandwich toaster until the cheese has melted.**
4. **Serve with the salad at once.**

Serving Suggestions: Add a glass of unsweetened fruit juice for a healthy lunch.

Storage: Not suitable for storage.

NUTRITIONAL ANALYSIS		Protein g	26.6	Fat g	13.2	Sodium g	0.9
PER PORTION		Carbohydrate g	47.4	Of which saturates g	0.6	Salt g	2.25
Energy kcal	414	Of which sugars g	13.2	Fibre g	1.2	Portion fruit and veg	2

Smoked Trout Sandwich
with Horseradish and Lamb's Lettuce

Serves: 1   **Prep:** 5 minutes

310kcal and 7.7g fat per portion

By using very low-fat cheese (only 4% fat) you won't need to use butter or any spread on your sandwich.

25g extra-light soft cheese

15g (1 level tbsp) horseradish sauce

72g (2 medium slices) granary bread

60g smoked trout

25g lamb's lettuce

50g cucumber, cut into wedges

1. **Mix the cheese with the horseradish and use to spread on one side of the bread.**
2. **Add the trout and lettuce, and put on the remaining bread.**
3. **Slice in half and serve with the cucumber wedges.**

Serving Suggestions: Add a pear and a glass of semi-skimmed milk.

Storage: You can store the sandwich in the fridge in an airtight container for 24 hours.

NUTRITIONAL ANALYSIS	Protein g	24.3	Fat g	7.7	Sodium g	1.3
PER PORTION	Carbohydrate g	36.2	Of which saturates g	2.2	Salt g	3.3
Energy kcal	310	Of which sugars g	6.8	Fibre g	3	Portion fruit and veg	1

Tuna and Sweetcorn Bagel (Dairy Free)

Serves: 1   **Prep:** 5 minutes
390kcal and 6.2g fat per portion

Often low-fat plain yogurt is used to mix with mayonnaise to reduce fat in recipe, but if you cannot tolerate dairy products you can substitute plain soya-based yogurt.

35g (1 rounded tbsp) plain soya yogurt

15g (1 level tbsp) reduced-fat mayonnaise (check the label to ensure dairy free)

100g canned tuna in spring water, drained

50g canned sweetcorn, drained

1 heaped tsp chopped parsley

80g (1 regular) bagel

Black pepper to season

1. Mix the yogurt and mayonnaise together, and stir in the tuna and sweetcorn.
2. Season with black pepper (do not add salt) and chopped parsley.
3. Warm or toast the bagel and slice in half. Fill with the tuna mix and serve.

Serving Suggestions: Add a few slices of cucumber and some cherry tomatoes.

Storage: The filling may be kept refrigerated for 2–3 days. Unsuitable for freezing.

NUTRITIONAL ANALYSIS		Protein g	38.2	Fat g	6.2	Sodium g	1.3
PER PORTION		Carbohydrate g	45.6	Of which saturates g	1.8	Salt g	3.25
Energy kcal	390	Of which sugars g	7	Fibre g	2.7	Portion fruit and veg	½

Turkey and Mango Mini-naan

Serves: 1   **Prep:** 5 minutes

445kcal and 8.3g fat per portion

Naan bread need not always be loaded with fat. Look for reduced-fat versions. These mini naan only contain 1.1g fat each.

100g (2) mini reduced-fat naan (e.g Sainsbury's BGTY)

14g (2 rounded tsp) low-fat spread (40% fat)

33g (1 rounded tbsp) mango chutney

40g (2 slices) turkey breast slices

30g lamb's lettuce

100g fresh mango slices or cubes

1. **Warm the naan bread, then carefully slice in half to make a pocket.**
2. **Spread with the low-fat spread and chutney, then tuck in a slice of turkey per naan.**
3. **Lastly add the lamb's lettuce.**
4. **Serve with the mango on the side.**

Serving Suggestions: A glass of plain lassi would complete your meal.

Storage: Not suitable for storage.

NUTRITIONAL ANALYSIS PER PORTION		Protein g	19.6	Fat g	8.3	Sodium g	0.9
		Carbohydrate g	72.6	Of which saturates g	1.7	Salt g	2.25
Energy kcal	445	Of which sugars g	31.5	Fibre g	5	Portion fruit and veg	1

Baked Potato with Curried Prawns

Serves: 1   **Prep:** 10 minutes   **Cook:** 60 minutes

375kcal and 8.5g fat per portion

A luscious prawn-and-cucumber filling for your baked potato, or use it in sandwiches instead.

120g (1 small) baking potato

50g extra-light soft cheese

15g (1 level tbsp) curry paste

20g (1) spring onion, finely chopped

40g cucumber, finely diced and drained in a sieve

100g cooked peeled prawns

30g salad leaves

4 cherry tomatoes

1. **Bake the potato in a hot oven (200°C/180°C Fan/GM6) until soft (about 1 hour) or cook in the microwave.**
2. **Meanwhile mix the soft cheese with the curry paste, onion and drained cucumber. When thoroughly mixed add the prawns.**
3. **Split open the potato and add the prawn mixture.**
4. **Serve with the salad leaves and tomatoes.**

Serving Suggestions: Replace the potato with 2 slices (72g) granary bread: 395kcal and 9.9g fat

Storage: The filling can be stored in the fridge for 24 hours provided the prawns are within use-by date. Not suitable for freezing.

NUTRITIONAL ANALYSIS		Protein g	31.7	Fat g	8.5	Sodium g	1.2
PER PORTION		Carbohydrate g	43.2	Of which saturates g	2.3	Salt g	3
Energy kcal	375	Of which sugars g	8.8	Fibre g	4.2	Portion fruit and veg	1

Main Course Salads

Asparagus and Egg Salad with Baby New Potatoes

Serves: 1   **Prep:** 10 minutes   **Cook:** 15 minutes

330kcal and 14.8g fat per portion

This is a great salad for summer when asparagus is in season, and the first new potatoes are in the shops. At other times of year, you can use green beans instead of asparagus.

160g baby new potatoes

1 large free-range egg

100g asparagus

30g (2 level tbsp) reduced-fat mayonnaise made with olive oil

Juice of half a lemon

30g (2 level tbsp) fat-free plain yogurt

4–5 leaves cos (romaine) lettuce, torn

1. Boil or steam the potatoes until just tender.
2. Hard boil the egg, then cool in running cold water. Slice into segments.
3. Steam the asparagus for 3–4 minutes until just tender.
4. Mix the mayonnaise with the lemon juice and yogurt.
5. Place the lettuce on the serving dish, and top with the potatoes, asparagus and egg.
6. Spoon over the dressing. Serve at once.

Serving Suggestions: Substitute green beans for the asparagus.

Storage: Not suitable for storage.

NUTRITIONAL ANALYSIS PER PORTION		Protein g	15.3	Fat g	14.8	Sodium g	0.3
		Carbohydrate g	33.5	Of which saturates g	2.9	Salt g	0.75
Energy kcal	330	Of which sugars g	7.9	Fibre g	2.3	Portion fruit and veg	1½

Tuna and Edamame Salad
with Avocado and Green Beans

Serves: 4   **Prep:** 10–15 minutes   **Cook:** 5 minutes

395kcal and 15.1g fat per portion

Enjoy all the benefits of soya, plus the chance to eat avocado, in this scrumptious salad.

200g frozen soya (edamame) beans

250g fine green beans

80g salad leaves

2 x 180g cans tuna in spring water, drained

200g (1 medium) hass avocado

Juice of half a lemon or lime

150g ciabatta, crisped in the oven and sliced

Chilli and Coriander Dressing (see page 241)

1. Boil the soya beans and steam the green beans for 5 minutes. Allow to cool.
2. Place the salad leaves in a large salad bowl.
3. Cut the green beans into short lengths and sprinkle these and the soya beans over the leaves.
4. Drain the tuna and break up the flakes slightly with a fork then add to the salad.
5. Peel and chop the avocado and sprinkle with the lemon juice to minimize it browning. Add to the salad.
6. Make the salad dressing by shaking all the ingredients together and pour over the salad.
7. Serve at once with crispy ciabatta.

Serving Suggestions: Make this up to take on a summer picnic, keeping the dressing separate until you are ready to serve.

Storage: Best eaten within a few hours of making,

NUTRITIONAL ANALYSIS PER PORTION		Protein g	29.9	Fat g	15.1	Sodium g	0.5
		Carbohydrate g	33.7	Of which saturates g	3.3	Salt g	1.25
Energy kcal	395	Of which sugars g	9.5	Fibre g	5.6	Portion fruit and veg	2

Pasta, Pesto and Chicken Salad

Serves: 2   **Prep:** 10–15 minutes   **Cook:** 12 minutes

440kcal and 12g fat per portion

If you like pesto then this is the salad for you. Although pesto is high in fat a little goes a long way, so you don't need much. Do make sure to measure it out accurately though.

120g fusilli or similar pasta

160g frozen sweetcorn

120g roast chicken, without the skin, roughly chopped

40g (2 medium) spring onions, chopped

30g (2 level tbsp) pesto

Few basil leaves, torn

160g cherry tomatoes, halved

1. Cook the pasta according to the packet instructions but without adding salt. In the last few minutes add and cook the sweetcorn. Drain well and allow to cool.

2. Place the pasta, sweetcorn, chicken and onions in a bowl. Stir in the pesto and basil leaves, and top with the cherry tomatoes.

3. Serve at once.

Serving Suggestions: Add a few salad leaves.

Storage: Can be refrigerated without the tomatoes for 24 hours. Not suitable for freezing.

NUTRITIONAL ANALYSIS PER PORTION	Protein g	30	Fat g	12	Sodium g	0.2
	Carbohydrate g	55.6	Of which saturates g	1.9	Salt g	0.5
Energy kcal	440	Of which sugars g	8.3	Fibre g	5	Portion fruit and veg	2

Pear and Feta Salad

Serves: 1   **Prep:** 5 minutes
390kcal and 11.5g fat per portion

A lovely salad for autumn when the pears are at their best. Rich in vitamin A and vitamin C, this salad also provides more than 2 portions of your 5 a day.

40g (half a bunch) watercress

170g (1 medium) conference pear

50g feta cheese

80g pomegranate seeds

2 tbsp Apple and Mint Dressing (see page 238)

40g (5-cm piece) French bread

1. **Roughly chop the watercress and place in a large salad bowl.**
2. **Wash and slice the pear into bite-size pieces and add to the bowl.**
3. **Crumble over the feta cheese and lastly sprinkle over the pomegranate seeds.**
4. **Serve with the dressing and use the bread to mop up the juices.**

Serving Suggestions: This also tastes delicious if you substitute the feta for pecan nuts. Remove 50g feta and add 25g pecans.

Storage: Not suitable for storage.

NUTRITIONAL ANALYSIS PER PORTION		Protein g	14.8	Fat g	11.5	Sodium g	0.7
		Carbohydrate g	61.5	Of which saturates g	7.4	Salt g	1.8
Energy kcal	390	Of which sugars g	40	Fibre g	8.4	Portion fruit and veg	2

Pearl Barley and Pomegranate Salad

Serves: 2 **Prep:** 5 minutes **Cook:** 45 minutes

175kcal and 3.6g fat per serving

Forget rice salad, and try fibre-rich nutty pearl barley. The pomegranate seeds look like rubies on the salad and taste fantastic. If they are out of season, use 2 clementines or 1 small orange cut into segments instead, catching any juice as you cut them for the salad.

70g pearl barley

2 tsp olive oil

75g pomegranate
  seeds

1 tbsp fresh parsley,
  chopped

Juice of 1 lemon

Black pepper

1. **Cook the pearl barley in plenty of water according to the packet instructions. It usually takes about 40 minutes to be tender.**
2. **Drain and rinse with cold water, and drain thoroughly.**
3. **Place the cooked barley in a serving bowl and stir through the olive oil, pomegranate seeds, parsley and lemon juice.**
4. **Season with black pepper.**
5. **Serve at room temperature.**

Serving Suggestions: Serve with grilled meat or fish, or as part of a salad meal with cold meats. Served with 100g ham: 223kcal and 4.4g fat.

Storage: Can store for 1 day only in the fridge, as there will be vitamin loss from the parsley and pomegranate.

NUTRITIONAL ANALYSIS PER PORTION	Protein g	4.2	Fat g	3.6	Sodium mg	0
	Carbohyrate g	31.8	Of which saturates g	0.5	Salt g	0
Kcal 175	Of which sugars g	4.9	Fibre g	5.9	Portion fruit and veg	½

Red Grape and Edam Salad with Pea Tops

Serves: 2   **Prep:** 5 minutes

277kcal and 13.4 Fat per serving

Look for pea tops in the supermarket. Like other new shoots, they are very high in vitamin C so you need to eat them very fresh to get the most out of them. Lamb's lettuce or Italian salad leaves would be a good alternative.

40–50g pea tops or salad leaves

1 medium red grapefruit

200g seedless red grapes, washed and halved

100g sliced Edam

1. Arrange the pea tops or salad leaves in a salad bowl.
2. Using a sharp knife, cut the peel and pith from around the grapefruit. Holding the grapefruit over the bowl to catch any juice, cut segments from the grapefruit.
3. Stir in the grapefruit segments and grapes.
4. Cut the sliced cheese into quarters and add to the salad.
5. Serve at once.

Serving Suggestions: Serve with a granary roll, or have with soup for a light meal.

Storage: Not suitable for storage.

NUTRITIONAL ANALYSIS PER PORTION		Protein g	15.5	Fat g	13.4	Sodium mg	506
		Carbohydrate g	25.3	Saturates	7.9	Salt equivalent g	1.3
Energy kcal	277	Of which sugars	25.3	Fibre g	2.9	Portion fruit and veg	2

Smoked Mackerel with Carrot and Currant Salad

Serves: 1   **Prep:** 5 minutes

360kcal and 14.6g fat per portion

Mackerel is an oily fish that provides essential omega-3 fatty acids, so this salad is a good one to add to your regular meals.

40g salad leaves

80g (about 4cm) cucumber, sliced

60g (1 small) carrot, grated

25g (1 tbsp) currants

Juice of 1 lime or half a lemon

½ tsp cumin seeds, toasted

60g smoked mackerel fillet, skinned and flaked

1 granary roll (50g)

1. **Place the salad leaves in a bowl and add the cucumber slices.**

2. **Mix together the carrot, currants, juice and cumin seeds in a bowl, and carefully mix in the smoked mackerel. Spoon on top of the salad leaves.**

3. **Serve straight away with the granary roll.**

Serving Suggestions: If you can't survive eating bread without spread, then use very low-fat spread: 2 level tsp (10g) very low-fat spread (20–25% fat) will add an extra 18kcal and 2g fat. 2 level tsp (10g) olive spread (60% fat) will add an extra 56kcal and 6.2g fat.

Storage: Best eaten with a few hours of serving. Not suitable for freezing.

NUTRITIONAL ANALYSIS		Protein g	16.9	Fat g	14.6	Sodium g	0.7
PER PORTION		Carbohydrate g	40	Of which saturates g	5.9	Salt g	1.75
Energy kcal	360	Of which sugars g	22	Fibre g	4.3	Portion fruit and veg	2

Summer Salad with Ciabatta

Serves: 2   **Prep:** 10 minutes
375kcal and 15.2g fat per serving

When summer fruit is at its height use it to add colour and vitamin C to your salads. The dressing with this salad is fat-free – look for balsamic glaze in the supermarket.

30g cos or other
  crunchy lettuce
40g (Half a bunch)
  watercress, rinsed
  and chopped
20g (2) spring onions,
  sliced
60g (4) cherry
  tomatoes, halved
80g (half) sweet red
  pepper, diced
50g reduced-fat
  feta cheese
20g walnuts, toasted
85g fresh
  blackcurrants or
  raspberries
1 tbsp balsamic glaze
140g ciabatta

1. Place the lettuce and watercress leaves in a salad bowl.
2. Add the spring onions, tomatoes and pepper.
3. Crumble over the feta, and add the walnuts and fruit.
4. Drizzle with balsamic glaze.
5. Serve at once with the bread.

Serving Suggestions: Replace the ciabatta and serve with 50g granary bread or rolls per serving: 280kcal, 12.3g fat.

Storage: Best served immediately to preserve vitamins and texture.

NUTRITIONAL ANALYSIS PER PORTION		Protein g	15	Fat g	15.2	Sodium mg	600
		Carbohydrate g	45.3	Of which saturates g	3.2	Salt g	1.5
Kcal	375	Of which sugars g	10.3	Fibre g	3.4	Portion fruit and veg	2

Tuna and Black Olive Bulghar Wheat Salad

Serves: 1   **Prep:** 5 minutes   **Cook:** 15 minutes

410kcal and 8.5g fat per portion

Bulghar wheat is a great source of fibre, and this salad provides one-third of your recommended 18g fibre per day. It is also low in GI so should keep the hunger pangs at bay.

50g bulghar wheat

120g canned tuna in
spring water

2 spring onions,
chopped

20g pitted sliced
black olives

40g (¼) green pepper,
diced

10g (1 rounded tsp)
sundried tomato
paste

Juice of half a lemon

1. Cook the bulghar wheat for 15 minutes in plenty of water, then drain well, and cool.
2. Mix together the tuna, onions, black olives and green pepper.
3. Mix together the tomato paste and lemon juice, and mix with the bulghar wheat.
4. Place the wheat in a bowl and stir in the other ingredients.
5. Serve immediately or chill for later use.

Serving Suggestions: Replace the sundried tomato paste for a similar quantity of pesto, and add a few basil leaves.

Storage: Can be chilled for 24 hours. Not suitable for freezing.

NUTRITIONAL ANALYSIS PER PORTION		Protein g	46.5	Fat g	8.5	Sodium g	0.9
		Carbohydrate g	37.3	Of which saturates g	1.1	Salt g	2.3
Energy kcal	410	Of which sugars g	4	Fibre g	6.8	Portion fruit and veg	1

Hot Garlicky King Prawn Salad

Serves: 1   **Prep:** 5 minutes   **Cook:** 20 minutes

300kcal and 8.2g fat per portion

If you've never had a hot salad before, this is the one to try: succulent, garlickly prawns with jewels of pomegranate.

150g salad potatoes, such as Charlotte

25g cos lettuce, roughly shredded

20g watercress, washed and dried

2 tsp olive oil

100g cooked peeled king prawns

1 clove garlic, crushed

30g pomegranate seeds

1 tbsp balsamic glaze

1. **Scrub the potatoes and boil or steam until just cooked. Allow to cool slightly.**
2. **Meanwhile arrange the lettuce and watercress on a serving plate.**
3. **Cut the cooked potatoes into quarters and place on the salad.**
4. **Heat the olive oil in a non-stick pan and quickly stir-fry the prawns and garlic for a couple of minutes.**
5. **Add the prawns to the salad and sprinkle over the pomegranate seeds.**
6. **Drizzle over the glaze and serve at once.**

Serving Suggestions: A 175ml glass of rosé or white wine is the perfect accompaniment – add 131kcal and 0g fat.

Storage: This really needs to be served warm, but you could make a cold version, which would keep a day in the fridge: just cool the potatoes and prawns before combining them with the salad ingredients.

NUTRITIONAL ANALYSIS PER PORTION		Protein g	22.6	Fat g	8.2	Sodium mg	0.5
		Carbohydrate g	35.5	Of which saturates g	1.6	Salt g	1.2
Energy kcal	300	Of which sugars g	9.1	Fibre g	3.6	Portion fruit and veg	1

Poultry

Apricot Chicken with Almonds and Pearl Barley

Serves: 4   **Prep:** 15 minutes   **Cook:** 40 minutes
485kcal and 12.9g fat per portion

A mildly spicy chicken dish topped with crunchy almonds and served with lemon- and parsley-scented pearl barley. The combination of pearl barley and apricots also makes this a high-fibre recipe.

140g pearl barley

1 tbsp rapeseed oil

160g (1 medium) red onion, sliced

3g (1 tsp) ground ginger

16g (2 level tbsp) ground coriander

500g skinless chicken breasts, cut into large cubes

200g dried apricots

500ml water ·

15g (1 level tbsp) cornflour

Juice of 1 lemon

Grated zest of 1 lemon

2 tbsp chopped fresh parsley

50g toasted almonds

1. **Cook the pearl barley according to the packet instructions.**
2. **Meanwhile heat the oil in a large non-stick pan and fry the onion for 5 minutes until softened.**
3. **Add the spices, chicken and apricots, then stir in the water.**
4. **Bring to simmering point and cook, covered, for 20–25 minutes, stirring occasionally.**
5. **Mix the cornflour with the lemon juice and add to the chicken. Cook for another few minutes to allow to thicken slightly.**
6. **When the pearl barley is cooked, drain well and stir in the lemon zest and parsley.**
7. **Sprinkle the almonds over the chicken to serve.**

Serving Suggestions: Serve with a green vegetable such as sugar snaps, steamed broccoli or courgettes. If you prefer to omit the almonds the nutrition per portion is: 416kcal and 5.8g fat.

Storage: Keep refrigerated for up to 2 days. Suitable for freezing.

NUTRITIONAL ANALYSIS		Protein g	39.7	Fat g	12.9	Sodium g	Trace
PER PORTION		Carbohydrate g	52.3	Of which saturates g	1.5	Salt g	trace
Energy kcal	485	Of which sugars g	20.4	Fibre g	14.4	Portion fruit and veg	1

Turkey Steaks with Crumb and Sundried Tomato Topping

Serves: 4   **Prep:** 5 minutes   **Cook:** 25–30 minutes
222kcal and 6.1g fat per portion

The ideal mid-week supper dish – simple and tasty, and can be prepared in advance! It is also full of flavour.

500g (ideally 4) turkey breast slices

20g (4 level tsp) pesto

75g white or half-and-half bread

40g sundried tomatoes in oil, drained

1 tbsp chopped fresh tarragon

Black pepper

1. **Preheat oven to 190°C/170°C Fan/GM5.**
2. **Lightly spray an ovenproof dish with cooking oil.**
3. **Place the turkey slices in the dish and spread with the pesto.**
4. **Place the bread and tomatoes in a food processor and blitz. Mix the tarragon with the breadcrumbs and grind over some pepper.**
5. **Spoon the crumb mixture over the turkey steaks, pressing down with a spoon.**
6. **Place the dish in the oven and cook for 25–30 minutes until the turkey is cooked through and the topping is golden brown.**

Serving Suggestions: Serve with Crushed New Potatoes with Herbs and Olive Oil (see page 215), sugar snaps and Pineapple Salsa (see page 245).

Storage: Can be prepared 1 day in advance and kept, refrigerated. Not suitable for freezing.

NUTRITIONAL ANALYSIS		Protein g	32.3	Fat g	6.1	Sodium g	0.2
PER PORTION		Carbohydrate g	9.6	Of which saturates g	0.7	Salt g	0.5
Energy kcal	222	Of which sugars g	0.5	Fibre g	0.7	Portion fruit and veg	0

Chicken and Parma Parcels

Serves: 2   **Prep:** 10 minutes   **Cook:** 30 minutes
228kcal and 6.1g fat per portion

The succulent filling in these parcels is kept in place by a wrapping of Parma ham. By baking the parcels in the oven there is no need to add unnecessary oil or fat.

250g (2 small) chicken breasts

40g frozen chopped spinach, thawed and well drained

Grated zest of half a lemon or lime

20g spring onions, finely chopped

50g extra-light soft cheese

½ tbsp chopped parsley

Grated nutmeg

56g (4 slices) Parma ham

1. Preheat oven to 190°C/170°C Fan/GM5.
2. Make a horizontal cut in the chicken breast to make a pouch in the flesh.
3. In a bowl mix together the spinach, lemon or lime zest, spring onions, soft cheese and parsley, and grate in nutmeg to taste.
4. Spoon half the mixture into the pouch and repeat with the other chicken breast.
5. Wrap 2 pieces of Parma ham around each chicken breast, securing them with a cocktail stick or string.
6. Lightly spray an ovenproof dish with oil, and bake in the oven for 25–30 minutes until the chicken is cooked through.
7. Serve hot.

Serving Suggestions: Serve with baby new potatoes, a green salad or the Okra with Tomatoes (page 218) and Citrus Couscous (page 213).

Storage: The parcels can be made in advance and kept in the fridge for up to 24 hours. Not suitable for freezing.

NUTRITIONAL ANALYSIS		Protein g	37.9	Fat g	6.1	Sodium g	0.7
PER PORTION		Carbohydrate g	1.4	Of which saturates g	2.3	Salt g	1.8
Energy kcal	228	Of which sugars g	1.3	Fibre g	0.9	Portion fruit and veg	0

Chicken and Peanut Stir-Fry

Serves: 4   **Prep:** 10 minutes   **Cook:** 10–15 minutes
314kcal and 14.9g fat per portion

Using a stir-fry sauce is an easy way of adding lots of flavour without a long list of individual spices. This recipe uses a ready-made peanut sauce, but you could use a lower-fat version if you prefer.

300g swede
150g green beans
2 tsp rapeseed oil
400g chicken breast, thinly sliced
75ml water
180g pack roasted peanut satay stir-fry sauce, e.g. Amoy

1. **Prepare the swede by peeling and cutting into very fine slices. Trim to make strips about 4cm in length.**

2. **Cut the beans into 2cm lengths and steam for 4–5 minutes until almost cooked. Remove from the heat.**

3. **Meanwhile heat the oil in a non-stick wok and quickly cook the chicken pieces for 5 minutes before adding the swede and the water. Continue to stir-fry for 3–4 minutes.**

4. **Stir in the cooked green beans and heat through for a minute or so.**

5. **Finally add the pack of stir-fry sauce, adding a little more water if required.**

6. **Serve at once.**

Serving Suggestions: Serve with rice, or noodles. Served without the peanut sauce and with soy sauce instead: 260kcal and 11.8g fat.

Storage: Not suitable for storage.

NUTRITIONAL ANALYSIS		Protein g	21.1	Fat g	14.9	Sodium g	0.9
PER PORTION		Carbohydrate g	25.1	Of which saturates g	2.5	Salt g	2.2
Energy kcal	314	Of which sugars g	12	Fibre g	3.4	Portion fruit and veg	1½

Chicken Fillets with Dill and Sundried Tomatoes

Serves: 2　**Prep:** 5 minutes　**Cook:** 25 minutes

234kcal and 11.3g fat per portion

This is a simple recipe that you can pop in the oven after work. It is great served with polenta (either ready-made or home-made).

240g chicken fillets

1 tsp dried dill or 1 tbsp chopped fresh dill

Black pepper

20g sundried tomatoes in oil, well drained

1. **Preheat oven to 190°C/170°C Fan/GM5.**
2. **Place the chicken fillets in a small ovenproof dish.**
3. **Sprinkle over the dill and generously grind over black pepper.**
4. **Chop the drained tomatoes and sprinkle over the chicken.**
5. **Cover with foil and place in the preheated oven for 20 minutes.**
6. **Remove from the oven and baste with the cooking juices, and return to the oven, uncovered, for another 5–10 minutes or until the chicken is cooked through.**
7. **Serve at once.**

Serving Suggestions: Serve with a green salad, or a mixture of green vegetables such as beans, mangetout, sugar snaps or broccoli. Served with 125g ready-made polenta: 324kcal and 11.7g fat.

Storage: This is not suitable for storage.

NUTRITIONAL ANALYSIS PER PORTION		Protein g	21.9	Fat g	11.3	Sodium g	0.6
		Carbohydrate g	11.6	Of which saturates g	1	Salt g	1.4
Energy kcal	234	Of which sugars g	1	Fibre g	0.1	Portion fruit and veg	0

Chicken Masala with Yogurt and Rice

Serves: 2   **Prep:** 15 minutes   **Cook:** 25 minutes
440kcal and 14.3g fat per serving

Measuring out oil and curry paste is important to keep this curry within your fat target.

4 tsp sunflower or
   vegetable oil
200g lean chicken
   breast, cut into
   cubes
1 small (60g) onion,
   finely chopped
1 tomato, skinned
   and chopped
1 level tbsp (18g) tikka
   masala curry paste
100ml water
100g low-fat plain
   yogurt
120g basmati rice

1. Preheat oven to 180°C/160°C Fan/GM4.
2. Heat 2 teaspoons of the oil in a non-stick pan and fry the chicken until just browned. Remove from the pan and keep warm.
3. Add 2 more teaspoons of oil to the pan and gently fry the onion until lightly browned.
4. Add the skinned, chopped tomato, the curry paste and water. Stir well to make a sauce, then take off the heat and add the yogurt.
5. Place the warm chicken in an ovenproof dish and pour over the sauce.
6. Cook, covered, in the preheated oven for 20–25 minutes until the chicken is cooked through.
7. Serve with the cooked rice.

Serving Suggestions: Serve with steamed spinach or green beans.

Storage: This will keep in the fridge for 2 days once cooked. Not suitable for freezing unless you stabilize the sauce by adding 1 tsp cornflour towards the end of cooking.

NUTRITIONAL ANALYSIS		Protein g	21.6	Fat g	14.3	Sodium mg	648
PER PORTION		Carbohydrate g	56.6	Of which saturates g	1.8	Salt g	1.6
Energy kcal	440	Of which sugars g	7.5	Fibre g	1	Portion fruit and veg	0

Chicken with Cajun Spices and Chickpeas

Serves: 4   **Prep:** 10 minutes   **Cook:** 20 minutes

265kcal and 7.7g fat per portion

An all-in-one meal high in essential vitamin A, which only needs the addition of couscous or bulghar wheat to make it complete. To save yourself preparation time, look for packs of frozen butternut squash.

2 tsp rapeseed oil

500g skinless chicken breasts, cubed

100g lean back bacon, trimmed of fat, diced

3 cloves garlic

6g (2 tsp) Cajun spices

300g prepared butternut squash, cut into large cubes.

400g can chickpeas in water, drained

200ml water

200g baby spinach, washed and drained

1. Heat the oil in a large non-stick pan, and gently fry the chicken and bacon for 5 minutes, stirring to prevent sticking.

2. Stir in the garlic and spices, and add the squash, chickpeas and water.

3. Bring to simmering point, then turn down the heat, cover and allow to cook gently for 15–20 minutes until the chicken is cooked through.

4. Add the spinach and allow to wilt before serving.

Serving Suggestions: Served with 50g (dry weight) couscous: 450kcal and 7.8g fat.

Storage: Can be stored in the fridge for up to 2 days. Not suitable for freezing.

NUTRITIONAL ANALYSIS PER PORTION	Protein g	39	Fat g	7.7	Sodium mg	500
	Carbohydrate g	9.7	Of which saturates g	1.9	Salt g	1.3
Energy kcal 265	Of which sugars g	2.1	Fibre g	6.7	Portion fruit and veg	2

Chicken, Fennel and Soya Bean Fricassée

Serves: 2 **Prep:** 10 minutes **Cook:** 20 minutes
507kcal and 12.4g fat per portion

This is a low-fat twist on a classic dish, which is served with brown rice. If you can't get soya beans you can substitute petits pois, or even sweetcorn.

250g skinless chicken breasts, cubed

200g fennel, cubed

1 small onion (60g) roughly chopped

¼ chicken stock cube

200ml semi-skimmed milk

1 large bay leaf

Few strips lemon rind

60g (dry weight) brown rice

Black pepper

30g (1 heaped tbsp) cornflour

30g (2 level tbsp) half-fat crème fraîche

160g frozen soya beans

1. Place the chicken, fennel and onion in a large non-stick saucepan.
2. Dissolve the stock cube in 50ml boiling water. Pour over the stock, milk and add the bay leaf and lemon rind.
3. Slowly bring to simmering point, then reduce the heat and poach gently for 15 minutes.
4. Meanwhile cook the brown rice.
5. Remove the bay leaf and lemon rind, and grind in some black pepper.
6. Mix the cornflour with the crème fraîche and stir into the fricassée. Increase the heat and allow mixture to bubble until just thickened.
7. Steam or microwave the soya beans and stir half into the mixture.
8. Drain the rice and divide between 2 serving plates, and add half the fricassée. Top with the remaining beans. Serve at once.

Storage: The fricassée alone (not rice) will keep in the fridge for up to 2 days.

NUTRITIONAL ANALYSIS		Protein g	47	Fat g	12.4	Sodium g	0.45
PER PORTION		Carbohydrate g	51.8	Of which saturates g	4.4	Salt g	1.0
Energy kcal	507	Of which sugars g	8.9	Fibre g	8.3	Portion fruit and veg	2

Chicken with Cherry Tomatoes and Leek Mash

Serves: 2   **Prep:** 10 minutes   **Cook:** 20–25 minutes

382kcal and 9.1g fat per portion

A delicious complete meal, in which the sweetness of the tomatoes is offset by the astringent balsamic vinegar. Tomatoes are rich in vitamin C and also lycopene, which becomes more readily available to the body when cooked.

2 tsp rapeseed oil

250g (2 small) chicken breasts

300g potatoes, peeled and quartered

100ml skimmed milk

140g (1 medium) leek, trimmed and finely sliced

1 tsp rapeseed oil

60g (1 small) red onion, finely chopped

1. Heat the oil in a non-stick frying pan and gently fry the chicken breasts for about 10 minutes on each side.

2. When the chicken is cooked, remove it from the pan and keep warm.

3. Meanwhile boil the potatoes in unsalted water.

4. Place the milk in a small saucepan and add the leek. Bring to simmering point and allow to cook gently for 10 minutes or until the leek is softened.

5. Add the remaining teaspoon of oil to the frying pan and fry the onion for 5 minutes until softened.

6. Stir in the tomatoes and turn up the heat. Cook until the tomatoes are breaking up, stirring frequently, for about 8 or so minutes.

NUTRITIONAL ANALYSIS	Protein g	36.4	Fat g	9.1	Sodium g	Trace
PER PORTION	Carbohydrate g	38.5	Of which saturates g	1.5	Salt g	Trace
Energy kcal	382	Of which sugars g	14.8	Fibre g	8.5	Portion fruit and veg	2

300g cherry
tomatoes, halved
2 tbsp balsamic
vinegar
5g (1 tsp) sugar
5g (1 tsp) <40% fat
spread
Black pepper

7. Add the balsamic vinegar and sugar, and boil very
briefly for a minute.
8. Drain the potatoes and mash with the milk in
which the leeks have been cooked, adding the
spread and some freshly ground black pepper.
When smooth, stir in the cooked leeks.
9. On a warm plate place half the leek mash in the
centre, add the chicken breast on top, and spoon
over the syrupy tomato sauce.
10. Serve at once.

Serving Suggestions: Add some steamed broccoli or
green beans.

Storage: Best served straight away. Not suitable
for freezing.

Coq au Vin

Serves: 4   **Prep:** 15 minutes   **Cook:** 30 minutes

275kcal and 13.5g fat per portion

A lower-fat take on a traditional favourite. A handy tip for peeling shallots is to pour boiling water over them for 1 minute to loosen the skin, then drain and peel.

1 tbsp olive oil

100g lean unsmoked back bacon, diced

140g (1 medium) leek, cut into 2–3cm chunks

200g small shallots, peeled

400g skinless, boneless chicken thighs, halved

200ml dry white wine

300ml water

2 bay leaves

Sprig of tarragon

200g baby mushrooms, left whole

15g (1 level tbsp) cornflour

Parsley, chopped

1. Heat the oil in a large non-stick casserole dish and fry the bacon for a few minutes to brown it.

2. Add the leek and shallots, and continue cooking to coat with the oil.

3. Now add the chicken, wine, water and herbs, and bring slowly to the boil.

4. Cover and reduce the heat, and allow to simmer gently for 20 minutes.

5. Now stir in the mushrooms and continue to cook for another 20–25 minutes until the chicken is tender and vegetables cooked.

6. Just before serving add the cornflour mixed with a little water and allow to thicken.

7. Serve hot with a sprinkling of chopped parsley.

Serving Suggestions: For an easy supper, serve with a crusty roll and green salad. Or try with Crushed New Potatoes with Herbs and Olive Oil (page 215): 410kcal and 17g fat.

Storage: May be frozen or will keep for a couple of days in the fridge.

NUTRITIONAL ANALYSIS PER PORTION						
	Protein g	26.7	Fat g	13.5	Sodium g	0.3
	Carbohydrate g	3.1	Of which saturates g	4.0	Salt g	0.75
Energy kcal	275	Of which sugars g	2.7	Fibre g	2.0	Portion fruit and veg	2

Coronation-style Turkey with Fresh Mango

Serves: 2　**Prep:** 5 minutes　**Cook:** 10 minutes
400kcal and 10g fat per portion

You can make this as hot or cool as you like by selecting a curry paste of your choice, be it korma or madras. The sauce is low in fat yet has a creamy texture, and can be made in advance for you just to add cooked turkey.

160g (1 medium) onion, finely chopped

1 tsp rapeseed oil

15g (1 level tbsp) curry paste

50g (1 heaped tbsp) mango chutney

50ml water

Juice of half a lemon

150g pot fat-free Greek yogurt

250g cooked skinless turkey, cut into pieces

150g mango cubes

Fresh coriander to garnish

1. Using a non-stick pan gently fry the onion in the oil for 5 minutes until starting to soften.

2. Stir in the curry paste, mango chutney and water, and continue to cook for 5 minutes or until the onion is soft.

3. Pour in the lemon juice and stir well.

4. Allow to cool for 5 minutes, then gradually stir in the yogurt.

5. Chill until you are ready to serve.

6. To serve, add the cooked turkey, fresh mango cubes and a sprinkling of chopped coriander.

Serving Suggestions: Serve with a baked sweet potato or rice, along with a leaf salad.

Storage: The sauce or the complete dish can be stored in the fridge for 2 days. Freezing not recommended.

NUTRITIONAL ANALYSIS		Protein g	47.5	Fat g	10	Sodium g	0.7
PER PORTION		Carbohydrate g	30	Of which saturates g	2.3	Salt g	1.8
Energy kcal	400	Of which sugars g	24.7	Fibre g	3.6	Portion fruit and veg	1

Duck with Water Chestnuts and Noodles

Serves: 1   **Prep:** 10 minutes   **Cook:** 10 minutes

455kcal and 9.2g fat per portion

For a special occasion why not treat yourself to duck? Look for skinless breast in the supermarket, which is actually very low in fat. You can, of course, replace the duck with chicken or turkey breast.

62g/1 nest (dry weight) egg noodles

2 tsp rapeseed oil

120g skinless duck breast, cut into fine slices

70g (½ small can) water chestnuts

40g (¼ medium) yellow pepper, finely sliced

40g (¼ medium) green pepper, finely sliced

1 spring onion, sliced

15ml oyster sauce

30ml dry sherry or Chinese wine

1. Soak the noodles in boiling water for 5 minutes until softened then drain and keep warm.
2. Heat the oil in a non-stick wok and fry the duck strips until just browned.
3. Add the water chestnuts, pepper and spring onion, and stir-fry for 3–4 minutes.
4. Mix together the oyster sauce and sherry, and pour into the wok, and mix around.
5. Combine the noodles with the duck and vegetables, and serve at once.

Serving Suggestions: Try with pak choi or mangetout instead of the peppers. Or try a ready-made stir-fry sauce, making sure it is low in fat.

Storage: Not suitable for storage.

NUTRITIONAL ANALYSIS PER PORTION		Protein g	33.6	Fat g	9.2	Sodium g	0.7
		Carbohydrate g	51.1	Of which saturates g	1.6	Salt g	1.75
Energy kcal	455	Of which sugars g	8.9	Fibre g	5.1	Portion fruit and veg	2

Greek Baked Chicken with Okra

Serves: 2   **Prep:** 10 minutes   **Cook:** 40–45 minutes

305kcal and 15.3g fat per portion

If you want to rekindle memories of that sun-soaked holiday, here is a dish to do it. The fresh oregano will transport you back to that Greek island, though the fat content of this is considerably lower than if eaten in Greece.

200g okra, trimmed

250g (3 medium) tomatoes, skinned and roughly chopped

250g skinless, boneless chicken thighs

1 tbsp chopped fresh oregano

Black pepper

100ml white wine

1 tbsp olive oil

1. **Preheat oven to 200°C/180°C Fan/GM6.**
2. **Place the trimmed okra in the base of a shallow ovenproof dish, and cover with the chopped tomatoes.**
3. **Place the chicken on top, and sprinkle over the oregano and black pepper.**
4. **Pour over the white wine and carefully spoon the oil over the chicken.**
5. **Place in the oven for 20 minutes, then remove and baste with the cooking juices.**
6. **Return to the oven and cook for another 15–20 minutes until the chicken is cooked through.**

Serving Suggestions: This can be served hot or at room temperature with rice and a green salad.

Storage: May be stored in the fridge for 1 day, and must be piping hot if reheated.

NUTRITIONAL ANALYSIS		Protein g	27.2	Fat g	15.3	Sodium g	Trace
PER PORTION		Carbohydrate g	7.1	Of which saturates g	4.1	Salt g	Trace
Energy kcal	305	Of which sugars g	6.3	Fibre g	5.3	Portion fruit and veg	2

Mexican Chicken in Chocolate

Serves: 2   **Prep:** 10 minutes   **Cook:** 30–40 minutes

330kcal and 6g fat per portion

If you like chilli with your chocolate you'll like this, and it may satisfy any chocolate cravings you have, too.

300g chicken breast fillets, skinned

80g (4) shallots, roughly chopped

50g sultanas

1 small chilli pepper, finely chopped

5g (1 rounded tsp) brown sugar

12g (2 rounded tsp) cocoa powder

15g (1 level tbsp) cornflour

¼ tsp ground cinnamon

30g (2 rounded tbsp) tomato purée

75ml red wine

100ml water

45g (1 rounded tbsp) reduced-fat crème fraîche

1. Preheat oven to 180°C/160°C Fan/GM4.
2. Place the chicken breasts in an ovenproof dish and sprinkle over the shallots, sultanas and chilli pepper.
3. Make the sauce by combining the sugar, cocoa, cornflour, and cinnamon with the tomato purée and wine.
4. Stir in the water and mix until smooth.
5. Pour into a saucepan and heat gently until the sauce thickens.
6. Remove from the heat, add the crème fraîche and pour over the chicken breasts.
7. Cover and cook for 25–35 minutes or until the chicken is cooked through.

Serving Suggestions: Serve with baked or mashed sweet potatoes, with a side salad. One portion served with 120g baked sweet potato, 40g leaf salad and 40g tomatoes: 480kcal and 6.8g fat.

Storage: Can be refrigerated for 2 days. Not suitable for freezing.

NUTRITIONAL ANALYSIS PER PORTION		Protein g	39.5	Fat g	6	Sodium g	0.2
		Carbohydrate g	22.8	Of which saturates g	3.1	Salt g	0.5
Energy kcal	330	Of which sugars g	22.2	Fibre g	1.5	Portion fruit and veg	1

Minty Chicken with Leek

Serves: 4 **Prep:** 10 minutes **Cook:** 20 minutes
190kcal and 4.9g fat per portion

The tangy sauce served with this chicken uses buttermilk, but you can use low-fat yogurt if you prefer. Either needs to be stabilized with a little cornflour to prevent it separating.

1 tbsp olive oil

300g leek, sliced into thin rounds

400g skinless chicken breast, cubed

284g carton buttermilk

10g (1 dsp) cornflour

1 heaped tsp hot horseradish sauce

Black pepper

1 tbsp chopped fresh mint

1. Heat the oil in a non-stick saucepan and gently fry the leek for 5 minutes.
2. Add the chicken, cover and cook gently for 10–15 minutes, adding a little water to prevent sticking if necessary.
3. Mix the buttermilk, cornflour and horseradish, and pour into the pan, stirring to make a sauce.
4. Allow the sauce to bubble gently and, when thickened, grind in some black pepper and stir in the mint.
5. Remove from the heat and serve at once.

Serving Suggestions: Serve with Crushed New Potatoes with Herbs and Olive Oil (see page 215) and broccoli.

Storage: Not suitable for freezing. Can be reheated after storing in the fridge for a maximum of 2 days.

NUTRITIONAL ANALYSIS		Protein g	27.7	Fat g	4.9	Sodium g	0.2
PER PORTION		Carbohydrate g	8.2	Of which saturates g	1.0	Salt g	0.5
Energy kcal	190	Of which sugars g	5.4	Fibre g	1.6	Portion fruit and veg	1

Oriental Mushrooms and Turkey with Rice Noodles

Serves: 2   **Prep:** 10 minutes   **Cook:** 10 minutes

410kcal and 6.9g fat per portion

Turkey and mushrooms make a super stir-fry. Using a non-stick pan is very helpful so you don't need to use much oil. If things start to stick, simply add a little water rather than more oil.

125g (dry weight) rice noodles

1 tbsp rapeseed oil

150g turkey breast strips

40g (4) spring onions, cut into 1-cm slices

150g mixed oriental mushrooms, sliced

1 red pepper, finely sliced

2 cloves garlic, crushed

1 tsp grated fresh ginger root

15ml (1 tbsp) soy sauce

15ml (1tbsp) oyster sauce

15ml (1 tbsp) dry sherry

1. Soak the rice noodles in boiling water for 5 minutes, then drain well.

2. Heat the oil in a non-stick wok or large frying pan and stir-fry the turkey breast for 5 minutes until cooked through. Remove from the pan and keep warm.

3. Add the spring onions, mushrooms and pepper, and stir-fry over a high heat for 3–4 minutes.

4. Add the garlic and ginger, and return the turkey to the pan, mixing all well together.

5. Mix the sauces and sherry, and pour into the wok, along with the noodles.

6. Stir through quickly and serve at once.

Serving Suggestions: A glass of chilled wine would be a great accompaniment.

Storage: Not suitable for storage.

NUTRITIONAL ANALYSIS PER PORTION		Protein g	26.3	Fat g	6.9	Sodium g	0.8
		Carbohydrate g	58.7	Of which saturates g	1	Salt g	2.0
Energy kcal	410	Of which sugars g	8.5	Fibre g	5.4	Portion fruit and veg	2

Turkey and Leek Risotto

Serves: 2   **Prep:** 5 minutes   **Cook:** 20 minutes

435kcal and 9.4g fat per portion

A great mid-week supper dish that uses many store-cupboard ingredients and is on the table within half an hour. Don't forget that stock can be very salty, and if you are using stock cubes you will only need about a quarter of one.

1 tbsp olive oil

140g (1 trimmed) leek, finely sliced

60g (2 small sticks) celery, diced

200g turkey breast, finely sliced

100g risotto rice

250ml chicken stock

40ml dry vermouth

160g sweetcorn, thawed if frozen

1 tbsp chopped parsley to serve

1. Heat the oil in a non-stick saucepan, and fry the leek and celery for 4–5 minutes until lightly browned.

2. Add the turkey and rice, and stir in 150ml of the stock, along with the vermouth.

3. Simmer gently for 15–20 minutes, stirring and adding more hot stock or some hot water as required.

4. When the rice is nearly tender, add the sweetcorn and heat through for another few minutes until hot.

5. Sprinkle over chopped parsley and serve at once.

Serving Suggestions: This is a complete meal, but you may like to add a few baby plum tomatoes, drizzled in balsamic glaze. Alternatively stir through 1 level tbsp (15g) of pesto just before serving: 490kcal and 12.9g fat.

Storage: Best served immediately.

NUTRITIONAL ANALYSIS PER PORTION							
	Protein g	32.1	Fat g	9.4	Sodium g	0.4
	Carbohydrate g	51	Of which saturates g	1.5	Salt g	1.0
Energy kcal	435	Of which sugars g	4.8	Fibre g	4.2	Portion fruit and veg	2

Sunflower Seed-coated Chicken with Yogurt Herb Salad

Serves: 4 **Prep:** 15 minutes **Cook:** 20 minutes
250kcal and 6.5g fat per portion

Instead of buying crumbed chicken pieces, which tend to be high in fat, why not make your own? They are not as difficult as you think.

70g white bread, made into breadcrumbs

1 tbsp chopped parsley

25g sunflower seeds

1 egg, beaten

400g skinless chicken breast fillet

For the dressing

100g low-fat plain yogurt

1 tsp sugar

Zest and 15ml of lemon or lime juice

1 tbsp chopped parsley

For the salad

150g cos lettuce, washed and torn into pieces

150g pomegranate seeds or chopped clementines

1. **Preheat oven to 190°C/170°C Fan/GM5 and spray a baking sheet with oil .**
2. **Mix together the breadcrumbs, parsley and sunflower seeds, and place in a large shallow bowl.**
3. **Place egg in a small shallow bowl.**
4. **Cut the chicken into strips and dip in the egg, then the breadcrumbs, and finally place on the baking sheet.**
5. **Repeat until all the chicken is coated, then bake for 20 minutes until cooked through.**
6. **Prepare the salad dressing by shaking all the ingredients together in a jar or container.**
7. **Place the lettuce in a salad bowl and pour over the dressing. Arrange the fruit on top.**
8. **Serve with the chicken pieces.**

Serving Suggestions: Serve with a crusty roll or small piece of ciabatta.

Storage: The dressing will keep in the fridge for 2–3 days. The cooked chicken pieces can be kept fo 2 days in the fridge and served cold. Not suitable for freezing.

NUTRITIONAL ANALYSIS PER PORTION	Protein g	30.8	Fat g	6.5	Sodium g	0.2
	Carbohydrate g	16.5	Of which saturates g	1.2	Salt g	0.5
Energy kcal 250	Of which sugars g	8.3	Fibre g	2.5	Portion fruit and veg	1

Turkey Burgers with Tomato and Red Onion Salad

Serves: 4   **Prep:** 10 minutes   **Cook:** 15 minutes

335kcal and 11.8g fat per portion

This is so easy, especially if you have a food processor, but don't worry if you haven't as the burger ingredients can be mixed together using a fork.

500g pack <5% fat turkey mince

2 cloves garlic, crushed

60g (1 small) onion, finely chopped

2 tbsp chopped parsley

Black pepper

½ tsp chilli flakes (optional)

Oil-mister

360g ripe tomatoes

60g (1 small) red onion

1 tbsp balsamic vinegar

1 tbsp olive oil

4 granary rolls (50g each)

1. Mix together the mince, garlic, onion, parsley, black pepper and chilli flakes in a food processor, or using a fork in a mixing bowl.

2. Shape the mixture into 4 burgers, using a little flour, if needed, to prevent stickiness.

3. Spray each burger lightly with oil and place under a preheated grill for 12–15 minutes, turning during cooking.

4. Meanwhile prepare the salad by finely slicing the tomato and onion, and layering on a plate. Drizzle over the vinegar and oil.

5. Halve the rolls and toast if desired.

6. When the burgers are cooked pop one in each roll and serve at once with the salad.

Serving Suggestions: Served with either the Spicy Harissa Dressing (page 250): 365kcal and 14.6g fat (for ¼ recipe), or the Pineapple Salsa (page 245): 358kcal and 11.9g fat (for ¼ recipe).

Storage: Not suitable for storage.

NUTRITIONAL ANALYSIS PER PORTION						
	Protein g	31	Fat g	11.8	Sodium g	0.4
	Carbohydrate g	25.4	Of which saturates g	3.0	Salt g	1
Energy kcal	335	Of which sugars g	6.5	Fibre g	2.6	Portion fruit and veg	1

Baked Chicken and Peaches Dressed with Lime and Sour Cream

Serves: 2   **Prep:** 5 minutes   **Cook:** 30 minutes
305kcal and 12.4g fat per serving

Look for reduced-fat sour cream, which has about 9g fat for every 100g, half the usual figure. To go lower still you can use fat-free plain yogurt, though the creamy texture of the dressing will be reduced.

250g (2 small) skinless
  chicken breasts
2 medium peaches
Zest and juice of
  1 lime
Black pepper
2 tbsp reduced-fat
  sour cream
½ tsp brown sugar

1. Preheat oven to 180°C/160°C Fan/GM4.
2. Place the chicken breasts in an ovenproof dish.
3. Cut the peaches into quarters and place around the chicken.
4. Finely grate the lime zest and keep for the dressing. Squeeze the lime and pour the juice over the chicken. Grind over some black pepper and cover with foil or a lid.
5. Place in the oven for 20 minutes, then uncover and baste with the cooking juices. Continue cooking for another 10 minutes or until the chicken in cooked through.
6. Meanwhile prepare the dressing by mixing the sour cream and zest with the sugar.

Serving Suggestions: Serve with boiled potatoes and, if in season, steamed courgettes or runner beans. Or try with plain couscous, peas and carrots.

Storage: This is best served straight away, although if you make up more of the dressing it will keep for a day or 2 in the fridge.

NUTRITIONAL ANALYSIS		Protein g	24.9	Fat g	12.4	Sodium g	0.6
PER PORTION		Carbohydrate g	24.9	Of which saturates g	2.9	Salt g	1.4
Energy kcal	305	Of which sugars g	12.9	Fibre g	2.2	Portion fruit and veg	1

Meat

Beef in Beer with Mustard Mash

Serves: 4   **Prep:** 15 minutes   **Cook:** 90–120 minutes

405kcal and 8.1g fat per portion

Many countries have their own version of beef in beer, so you can use whichever ale you fancy. This one uses stout, which complements the mushrooms and steak very well.

30g (1 heaped tbsp) flour	1. Preheat oven to 160°C/140°C Fan/GM3.
1 tsp dried mixed herbs	2. Place the flour, herbs and pepper in a large plastic bag.
Black pepper	3. Drop the cubes of beef into the bag and shake to coat the meat with the seasoned flour.
500g extra-lean stewing steak, cut into cubes	4. Place the shallots and seasoned meat in a large casserole and add the stout and mushroom ketchup or Worcestershire sauce.
300g small shallots, peeled	5. Stir, cover and gradually bring to simmering point on the hob, stirring occasionally.
350ml stout	6. Transfer to the oven and cook for 1 hour, then add the mushrooms.
1 tbsp mushroom ketchup (or Worcestershire sauce)	7. Cook for another 20–30 minutes until the meat is tender.
200g button mushrooms	8. Make the mustard mash by boiling the potatoes until just soft. Drain and mash with the milk until smooth and creamy, then stir in the wholegrain mustard.
700g potatoes	
50ml semi-skimmed milk	
25g wholegrain mustard	

Serving Suggestions: Add some freshly cooked cabbage or spinach to perfect your meal.

Storage: The casserole can be stored in the fridge for 2–3 days and is suitable for freezing.

NUTRITIONAL ANALYSIS PER PORTION		Protein g	35.6	Fat g	8.1	Sodium g	0.2
		Carbohydrate g	43.4	Of which saturates g	2.7	Salt g	0.5
Energy kcal	405	Of which sugars g	10.3	Fibre g	4.5	Portion fruit and veg	1

Venison with Plums and Port

Serves: 4 **Prep:** 5 minutes **Cook:** 120 minutes

315kcal and 3.2g fat per portion

This venison casserole is perfect for a special occasion, and can be made in advance and frozen. Venison is naturally low in fat and a great source of iron.

700g diced venison

320g (2 medium) red onions, quartered

300g plums, stoned and quartered

50g chopped prunes

½ tsp ground cinnamon

Pinch of ground cloves

120ml port

150ml water

15g (1 level tbsp) cornflour

1. **Preheat oven to 160°C/140°C Fan/GM3.**
2. **Place all the ingredients except the cornflour in an ovenproof casserole.**
3. **Cover and place the casserole in the oven and cook for 1½ hours.**
4. **Remove from the oven, and stir in the cornflour, mixed with a little water.**
5. **Return to the oven for another 20–30 minutes until the meat is tender.**

Serving Suggestions: Serve with Leek and Mustard Mash (page 217) and fresh cabbage or green beans.

Storage: This casserole will keep in the fridge for 2–3 days in an airtight container. It is also suitable for freezing.

NUTRITIONAL ANALYSIS PER PORTION		Protein g	40.6	Fat g	3.2	Sodium g	0.1
		Carbohydrate g	24.2	Of which saturates g	1.4	Salt g	0.2
Energy kcal	315	Of which sugars g	18.9	Fibre g	3.0	Portion fruit and veg	1

Beef with Sweet Chestnuts

Serves: 4   **Prep:** 10 minutes   **Cook:** 90–120 minutes

275kcal and 10.5g fat per portion

Look for vacuum-packed or frozen sweet chestnuts to make this dish. Also choose your passata carefully, opting for the unsalted if possible.

500g lean braising steak, cut into cubes

160g (1 medium) onion, finely chopped

3 cloves garlic, left whole

100g frozen or vacuum-packed chestnuts

5g (1 tsp) smoked hot paprika

Black pepper

400g passata

140ml (4 rounded tbsp) half-fat sour cream

Parsley

1. Preheat oven to 170°C/150°C Fan/GM3.
2. Place the beef, onion, garlic and chestnuts in a large ovenproof casserole.
3. Sprinkle over the paprika and pepper, and stir to distribute evenly.
4. Pour in the passata and cover.
5. Place in the oven and cook, stirring once or twice during cooking for 1½–2 hours until the meat is tender. During the last 20 minutes or so you can remove the lid to allow the sauce to thicken. Alternatively crush some of the chestnuts before serving.
6. Serve with a rounded tablespoon of sour cream per portion and a sprinkling of chopped parsley.

Serving Suggestions: A green vegetable such as broccoli or green beans is an ideal accompaniment. Why not place some potatoes in the oven to bake at the same time?

Storage: Without the addition of the sour cream the stew can be refrigerated for a few days or frozen.

NUTRITIONAL ANALYSIS PER PORTION		Protein g	29.2	Fat g	10.5	Sodium g	Trace
		Carbohydrate g	16.4	Of which saturates g	4.6	Salt g	Trace
Energy kcal	275	Of which sugars g	7.4	Fibre g	2.3	Portion fruit and veg	1

Chilli con Carne

Serves: 4 or 6   **Prep:** 15 minutes   **Cook:** 30–40 minutes
315kcal and 12.6g fat per ¼ recipe
210kcal and 8.4g fat per ⅙ recipe

An old favourite that is made without added oil. You can omit the jalapeños if you don't like them, and add fresh chilli or chilli powder instead.

500g extra-lean
  minced beef
160g (1 medium) onion,
  finely sliced
2 cloves garlic,
  crushed
30g jalapeño
  peppers, chopped
400g can chopped
  tomatoes
30g (2 tbsp) tomato
  paste
400g can kidney
  beans in water,
  drained and rinsed
2 tbsp chopped fresh
  coriander

1. Place the minced beef in a large non-stick saucepan and heat gently, breaking up the meat with a wooden spoon.

2. As the meat starts to brown and release juices and fat, add the onion and garlic, and gently fry for 7–8 minutes.

3. When the meat is browned all over add the jalapeños, tomatoes and tomato paste, and bring to the boil.

4. Add the kidney beans, cover and simmer for 20–25 minutes until the meat is cooked and the sauce is starting to thicken.

5. Serve sprinkled with the coriander.

Serving Suggestions: Serve with a baked sweet potato or rice and a green salad. A 130g sweet potato provides 109kcal and 0.3g fat.

Storage: Can be frozen for later use. Refrigerate in an airtight container for 2–3 days.

Serves 4

NUTRITIONAL ANALYSIS PER PORTION		Protein g	33.4	Fat g	12.6	Sodium g	0.4
		Carbohydrate g	17.8	Of which saturates g	5.3	Salt g	1
Energy kcal	315	Of which sugars g	8.8	Fibre g	5.1	Portion fruit and veg	2

Serves 6

NUTRITIONAL ANALYSIS PER PORTION		Protein g	22.3	Fat g	8.4	Sodium g	0.3
		Carbohydrate g	11.9	Of which saturates g	3.5	Salt g	0.75
Energy kcal	210	Of which sugars g	5.5	Fibre g	3.4	Portion fruit and veg	2

Fresh Pea and Ham Risotto

Serves: 4   **Prep:** 5 minutes   **Cook:** 20–25 minutes
400kcal and 9.2g fat per serving

This simple summer risotto calls for a trip to the deli counter to ask for thick-cut ham. You should ask for 2 slices (to make 200g), which you can then dice at home. When fresh peas are not in season use frozen; allow to thaw and just stir in at the end.

1 tbsp olive oil

4 spring onions, cut into 1-cm slices

300g risotto rice

500ml vegetable stock

200g thick-cut ham

300g shelled fresh peas (or about 750g unshelled)

40g (4 tbsp) grated parmesan

1. Heat the oil in a shallow non-stick pan and gently fry the spring onions until they are becoming a little transparent.
2. Add the risotto rice and stir around to prevent sticking. Stir in 300ml of the hot vegetable stock.
3. Allow to simmer, stirring frequently, and gradually add the remaining hot stock.
4. Meanwhile dice the ham and, if required, shell the peas.
5. When the rice is almost cooked through (about 15–20 minutes) stir in the peas and ham, and, if necessary, add more stock.
6. Allow the peas to cook through.
7. Serve with 1 tablespoon of parmesan per person.

Serving Suggestions: Add a few cherry tomatoes for colour and additional vitamin C.

Storage: Not suitable for storing.

NUTRITIONAL ANALYSIS PER PORTION		Protein g	22.2	Fat g	9.2	Sodium mg	624
		Carbohydrate g	56	Of which saturates g	2.9	Salt g	1.6
Energy kcal	400	Of which sugars g	2	Fibre g	3.1	Portion fruit and veg	1

Gammon with Sweet-and-sour Shallots

Serves: 2   **Prep:** 5 minutes   **Cook:** 20 minutes

310kcal and 12g fat per portion

Lean gammon tastes wonderful with this sticky sauce. Although it is not high in fat, gammon can be very salty, so look out for this on the label when you are choosing your meat.

150g shallots, finely chopped

15g muscovado sugar

1 tbsp balsamic vinegar

70ml freshly squeezed orange juice

300g lean smoked gammon steak, cut in half (or 2 x 150g steaks)

1. Place the shallots, sugar, vinegar and orange juice in a saucepan and allow the sauce to come to the boil, then reduce the heat.

2. Let the sauce simmer slowly stirring occasionally until the shallots are cooked and the sauce is starting to caramelize – about 15 minutes. If the sauce starts to stick add a little more orange juice.

3. Meanwhile grill the gammon until it is tender and cooked through – 5–8 minutes each side, depending on its thickness.

4. Serve the gammon with the shallots.

Serving Suggestions: Serve with mashed potatoes and a green vegetable.

Storage: The sauce will keep in the fridge for 2 days in an airtight container.

NUTRITIONAL ANALYSIS		Protein g	37.2	Fat g	12	Sodium g	1.8
PER PORTION		Carbohydrate g	14.4	Of which saturates g	4.5	Salt g	4.5
Energy kcal	310	Of which sugars g	14.4	Fibre g	0.7	Portion fruit and veg	½

Grilled Teriyaki Pork with Orange

Serves: 2   **Prep:** 5 minutes   **Cook:** 30 minutes inc marianade
175kcal and 4.2g fat per serving

A really simple, quick supper dish that is also great if you are barbecuing outside in the summer. Teriyaki, like other soy sauces, is very salty, so don't be tempted to add too much.

250g pork fillet

1 large orange

2 tbsp teriyaki sauce

1 bunch (80g)
   watercress to
   serve

1. Cut the pork fillet into slices about 1-cm thick.
2. Grate the orange rind, then cut the orange in half. Put one half aside.
3. Squeeze the other half-orange and mix the juice and grated rind with the teriyaki sauce. Pour over the pork fillet. Cover and allow to marinate for a minimum of 20 minutes.
4. Cook the pork on a barbecue or hot grill and serve garnished with the segments from the saved orange and the watercress.

Serving Suggestions: Serve with grilled polenta or couscous salad. Served with 250g ready-made grilled polenta: 295kcal and 5.5g fat.

Storage: The pork can be marinated overnight in the fridge. Otherwise unsuitable for longer storage.

NUTRITIONAL ANALYSIS PER PORTION			Protein g	26	Fat g	4.2	Sodium mg	964
			Carbohydrate g	9.1	Of which saturates g	0	Salt g	2.4
Energy kcal		175	Of which sugars g	9	Fibre g	1.6	Portion fruit and veg	½

Home-made Burgers with Spicy Potato Wedges

Serves: 4   **Prep:** 5 minutes   **Cook:** 30–40 minutes
360kcal and 12.1g fat per portion

Burgers made with lean mince are not high in fat and are delicious. These contain a little sundried tomato paste, but you could replace this with some mixed herbs, or add chilli paste if you like your burgers hot.

800g potatoes, e.g. King Edward
Oil-mister
1 tsp Cajun spices
500g extra-lean minced beef (<5% fat)
30g (1 level tbsp) sundried tomato paste
4 (40g) spring onions

1. Preheat oven to 200°C/180°C Fan/GM6.
2. Scrub the potatoes and cut lengthwise to make 6–8 wedges.
3. Place the potatoes on a non-stick baking sheet, and spray lightly with oil. Sprinkle over the Cajun spices and place in the oven for 30–40 minutes.
4. In a food processor mix together the mince, tomato paste and spring onions.
5. Make the mince mixture into 4 burgers, using a little flour if sticky.
6. Slowly cook the burgers in a non-stick saucepan, or grill until the centre of the burgers is cooked through and no longer pink. Alternatively place in the oven with the wedges and bake.
7. Serve with wedges and salad.

Serving Suggestions: Try with Raspberry Salsa (page 248): 393kcal and 12.4g fat.

Storage: Not suitable for storage.

NUTRITIONAL ANALYSIS PER PORTION		Protein g	30.5	Fat g	12.1	Sodium g	0.2
		Carbohydrate g	34.2	Of which saturates g	3.3	Salt g	0.5
Energy kcal	360	Of which sugars g	1.4	Fibre g	2.7	Portion fruit and veg	0

Jambalaya

Serves: 4   **Prep:** 10 minutes   **Cook:** 25 minutes

500kcal and 11.4g fat per portion

Jambalaya comes from the deep south of the US and is a delicious mixture of poultry and fish with spicy sausage. This version uses chorizo sausage to provide the oil, in which the chicken cooks, and impart a delicious spiciness.

300g (dry weight) long-grain rice

75g chorizo sausage, cut into cubes

200g skinless chicken breast, cut into small pieces

250g (1 large) green pepper, sliced

250g (1 large) red pepper, sliced

3 cloves garlic

250g (2 large) tomatoes, skinned and roughly chopped

2 tsp blackened Cajun spices

180g cooked peeled jumbo king prawns

1. Cook the rice according to the packet instructions.

2. Place the chorizo in a large non-stick sauté pan and gently heat to release the fat in the sausage, stirring often.

3. Add the chicken and cook for 5 minutes.

4. Add the peppers and garlic, and continue cooking over a low heat for another 5 minutes before adding the tomatoes and spices.

5. Let the mixture bubble away for another 10 minutes, stirring occasionally.

6. Add the prawns to the mixture while you drain the rice, saving a few prawns for decoration.

7. Combine the rice with the rest of the mixture and stir to coat all the rice with the juices.

8. Serve at once.

Serving Suggestions: Add a green salad or peas.

Storage: Can be kept in the fridge for 1 day, and reheated in a microwave oven until piping hot. Not suitable for freezing.

NUTRITIONAL ANALYSIS	Protein g	32	Fat g	11.4	Sodium g	0.5
PER PORTION	Carbohydrate g	71.6	Of which saturates g	3.1	Salt g	1.3
Energy kcal 500	Of which sugars g	6.6	Fibre g	3	Portion fruit and veg	1½

Lamb and Coconut with Noodles

Serves: 2   **Prep:** 10 minutes   **Cook:** 25 minutes
455kcal and 13.4g fat per portion

A little coconut goes a long way, so although it is high in fat, by measuring it out carefully you can enjoy the taste of coconut without adding too many calories or grams of fat.

200g lean diced lamb

50g (5) spring onions, sliced

160g (1 medium) green pepper

160g (1 medium) yellow pepper

25g creamed coconut

200ml boiling water

1 tsp grated ginger

2 cloves garlic, crushed

1 lemon grass stalk finely chopped

125g (2 nests) thick egg noodles

2 tbsp roughly chopped coriander

1. **Place the lamb, onions and peppers in a non-stick saucepan.**
2. **Dissolve the creamed coconut in the boiling water and pour into the casserole.**
3. **Stir in the ginger, garlic and lemon grass.**
4. **Cover and gently cook on the hob for 20–25 minutes, stirring occasionally.**
5. **Cook the noodles according to the packet instructions.**
6. **When the lamb is tender stir in the coriander and serve at once with the noodles.**

Serving Suggestions: Steam 2 heads of roughly chopped pak choi.

Storage: Can be frozen or refrigerated for 2 days.

NUTRITIONAL ANALYSIS		Protein g	31.3	Fat g	13.4	Sodium g	0.4
PER PORTION		Carbohydrate g	52.9	Of which saturates g	9.1	Salt g	1
Energy kcal	455	Of which sugars g	9.9	Fibre g	4.6	Portion fruit and veg	1

Lamb and Apricot Tagine

Serves: 4 **Prep:** 15 minutes **Cook:** 60–90 minutes
380kcal and 11.2g fat per portion

This Moroccan favourite uses very lean diced lamb such as Sainsbury's Be Good to Yourself diced lamb. Apricots add sweetness and texture to the recipe as well as fibre and vitamin A.

2 tbsp olive oil

600g very lean lamb, diced

2 red onions, sliced

3 cloves garlic, crushed

1 tbsp cumin seeds, crushed

1 tsp ground cinnamon

4 kaffir lime leaves

400ml water

45g (3 level tbsp) tomato purée

1 small red chilli, seeded and finely chopped

250g dried apricots

150g low-fat plain yogurt

2 tbsp chopped coriander

1. In a large heavy-bottomed pan or casserole, heat 1 tablespoon of the oil and gently fry the lamb until lightly browned.

2. Remove the lamb and add the remaining olive oil, onions and garlic, and fry until the onion is softened.

3. Add the spices and lime leaves and stir around, adding a little water if needed to prevent burning.

4. Return the lamb to the pan along with the water, tomato purée, chilli and apricots.

5. Stir well. Bring slowly to simmering point. Cover and cook over a gentle heat for 1–1½ hours or until the lamb is cooked through and tender. Add more water during cooking if necessary.

6. Remove the lime leaves and serve with the plain yogurt and chopped coriander.

Serving Suggestions: Serve with couscous and a green salad. 30g (dry weight) portion of couscous with 1 serving tagine: 480kcal and 11.3g fat.

Storage: Can be frozen or kept in the fridge for 2–3 days in an airtight container. Reheat until piping hot.

NUTRITIONAL ANALYSIS PER PORTION		Protein g	37.1	Fat g	11.2	Sodium g	Trace
		Carbohydrate g	32.5	Of which saturates g	3.1	Salt g	Trace
Energy kcal	380	Of which sugars g	30.3	Fibre g	5.5	Portion fruit and veg	2

Maple Lamb with Butternut Squash

Serves: 4   **Prep:** 10 minutes   **Cook:** 105 minutes

292kcal and 10.4g fat per portion

This delicious lamb casserole will just cook away while you do something else.

500g very lean lamb, cut into cubes

300g red onions (2 medium), sliced

2 cloves garlic, crushed

500g butternut squash, cubed

200g carrots, trimmed and cut into chunks

1 tbsp ground coriander

1 tbsp maple syrup

2 tbsp (50g) tomato purée

500ml water

15g (1 level tbsp) cornflour

Black pepper

Parsley

1. Preheat oven to 150°C/130°C Fan/GM2.
2. Place the lamb, onions, garlic, squash and carrots in a large casserole dish.
3. Mix the coriander with the maple syrup and tomato purée, and gradually stir in the water.
4. Pour over the lamb and vegetables. Season with black pepper.
5. Cover and place in the oven to cook for 1¼ hours, then check and stir.
6. Continue cooking until the meat is tender, up to another 30 minutes.
7. Garnish with chopped parsley and serve.

Serving Suggestions: Serve with hot vegetables such as broccoli and mangetout and a baked potato.

Storage: Suitable for freezing or can be kept in the fridge for 2 days.

NUTRITIONAL ANALYSIS PER PORTION		Protein g	28.7	Fat g	10.4	Sodium mg	trace
		Carbohydrate g	24	Of which saturates g	0.1	Salt g	0.1
Energy kcal	292	Of which sugars g	16.9	Fibre g	5.7	Portion fruit and veg	1

Marinated Lamb
with Crushed Potatoes

Serves: 2   **Prep:** 10 minutes + 30 marinating   **Cook:** 10–12 minutes
335kcal and 13.8g fat per portion

If you are barbecuing, here is one to try – tender lean lamb steaks with a honey-and-spice dressing skewered with courgettes and mushrooms.

200g extra-trimmed
lamb steak

20ml lemon juice
(juice of half a
lemon)

1 tsp ground ginger

1 tsp ground
cinnamon

16g (2 tsp) runny
honey

100g baby
mushrooms, wiped

100g (1 medium)
courgette, cut into
thick slices

Fresh bay leaves

250g new potatoes,
scrubbed

1 tbsp olive oil

Black pepper

Fresh mint

1. Cut the lamb steaks into 2-cm cubes.
2. Place the juice, spices and honey in a bowl, and mix together. Add the lamb, cover and marinate for at least 30 minutes, preferably a few hours.
3. When you are ready to cook, preheat the grill or barbecue and thread the lamb, mushroom, courgette and bay leaves onto skewers.
4. Cook for 4–5 minutes each side.
5. Meanwhile boil or steam the potatoes until tender.
6. Drain the potatoes and press gently with a potato masher. Place in a serving dish and drizzle over the oil. Grind plenty of black pepper on top and sprinkle over chopped mint.
7. Serve the lamb with the crushed potatoes.

Serving Suggestions: Try this with Greek Peas with Leeks and Mint (see page 216).

Storage: The lamb can be marinated for up to 24 hours in advance. The cooked dish is not suitable for storage.

NUTRITIONAL ANALYSIS PER PORTION	Protein g	23.6	Fat g	13.8	Sodium g	Trace
	Carbohydrate g	30.5	Of which saturates g	1	Salt g	Trace
Energy kcal	335	Of which sugars g	10.2	Fibre g	3.4	Portion fruit and veg	1

Pork Chop in Citrus Sauce

Serves: 1   **Prep:** 5 minutes   **Cook:** 20–25 minutes
325kcal and 10.9g fat per portion

A chunky but lean pork chop cooked in fresh orange juice makes an easy supper dish for one.

170g lean pork chop, trimmed of any visible fat

1 shallot, finely chopped

60ml freshly squeezed orange juice (about 1 small orange)

Zest of 1 lime

3–4 basil leaves

1. Place the chop in a small non-stick pan and cook for 5 minutes, turning once to allow the chop to brown.
2. Stir in the shallot and cook for a couple of minutes.
3. Pour in the orange juice, grated lime zest and basil leaves.
4. Allow to come to simmering point then cover; reduce the heat and cook gently for 20 minutes or until the chop is cooked through.
5. Serve at once.

Serving Suggestions: Serve with mashed potato, pasta or couscous. A smaller chop (130g) would provide 250kcal and 8.3g fat.

Storage: Not suitable for storage.

NUTRITIONAL ANALYSIS		Protein g	54	Fat g	10.9	Sodium g	0.1
PER PORTION		Carbohydrate g	2.3	Of which saturates g	3.7	Salt g	0,2
Energy kcal	325	Of which sugars g	2.3	Fibre g	0	Portion fruit and veg	0

Moussaka

Serves: 4   **Prep:** 35 minutes   **Cook:** 45 minutes
326kcal 14.8g fat per serving

Who says you need to fry aubergines to make moussaka? Oven bake them with
a light spraying of oil and you can still enjoy this classic dish.

2 medium aubergines,
thinly sliced

Oil spray

400g extra-lean
minced beef

1 medium onion, finely
chopped

1 clove garlic,
crushed

1 tsp ground
cinnamon

140g can tomato
purée

150ml red wine

200ml beef stock

1. Preheat oven to 180°C/160°C Fan/GM4.
2. Place the aubergine slices on a baking sheet and
   lightly spray with oil. Place in the preheated oven
   for 20–25 minutes turning once, until the
   aubergines are just softening. Remove from the
   heat and cool. Turn up the oven to 190°C/170°C
   Fan/GM5.
3. Meanwhile, gently brown the mince and onion in a
   large non-stick saucepan. Cook until the meat is
   browned, stirring to break up the mince.
4. Add the crushed garlic, cinnamon and the tomato
   purée and stir well.
5. Pour in the wine and beef stock, and simmer for
   25 minutes, stirring occasionally, adding a little
   water if the mixture is too thick.

NUTRITIONAL ANALYSIS	Protein g	30.5	Fat g	14.8	Sodium mg	364
PER PORTION	Carbohydrate g	13.1	Of which saturates g	5.5	Salt g	0.9
Kcal	326	Of which sugars g	11.9	Fibre g	4.0	Portion fruit and veg	1½

2 medium eggs
284ml carton
 buttermilk
Nutmeg

6. In a large flat, ovenproof dish, spread a layer of
   the mince sauce followed by a layer of
   aubergines. Use up the sauce and aubergines in
   this way.
7. Beat the eggs with the buttermilk and pour over
   the moussaka.
8. Grate plenty of nutmeg on top.
9. Bake for 35–45 minutes until the aubergines are
   soft and the topping just browning.
10. Serve with rice or bread and green vegetables or
    a salad of coloured leaves.

Serving Suggestions: When served with 40g (dry
weight) basmati rice and 90g green beans: 489kcal and
15.2g fat.

Storage: Will keep in the fridge for 2–3 days.

Old-fashioned Steak and Kidney Cobbler

Serves: 4   **Prep:** 20 minutes   **Cook:** 70 minutes

453kcal and 15.6g fat per portion

By using lean beef you can have this traditional favourite that you may have thought was forbidden while you were on a diet! If you don't like kidney, just replace it with lean beef.

Ingredients	Method
450g pack steak-and-kidney, e.g. Waitrose	1. Preheat oven to 160°C/140°C Fan/GM3.
15g (1 level tbsp) flour	2. Coat the meat by placing in a bag with the flour and shaking.
200g small shallots, peeled and left whole	3. Place the meat in a large ovenproof pan that can also be used on the hob.
2 bay leaves	4. Add the shallots, bay leaves and stock.
300ml beef stock or 300ml water with half a stock cube	5. Bring the mixture gently to the boil, stirring occasionally.
225g flour	6. Cover and put in the oven for 45–50 minutes.
5g (1 heaped tsp) baking powder	7. Meanwhile make the scone topping by mixing the flour and baking powder with the sage, and rubbing in the olive spread.
	8. Stir the milk into the dry scone ingredients to make a soft but not sticky dough.

NUTRITIONAL ANALYSIS	Protein g	31.3	Fat g	15.6	Sodium g	0.5
PER PORTION	Carbohydrate g	47	Of which saturates g	5.2	Salt g	1.3
Energy kcal	453	Of which sugars g	3.8	Fibre g	3.1	Portion fruit and veg	½

1 tsp dried sage
30g olive spread
125ml skimmed milk
200g chestnut
   mushrooms,
   quartered
Parsley

9. Using a little extra flour, roll out the mixture to around 2cm thickness and cut 8 scones from the dough. Keep to one side.

10. Remove the stew from the oven and stir in the mushrooms. Turn the oven up to 200°C/180°C Fan/GM6.

11. If the sauce is a little thin, mix a tablespoon of cornflour with a little water and stir into the stew at this point.

12. Carefully arrange the scones on top of the stew and return to the hot oven for 15–20 minutes until the scones have risen.

13. Serve at once, sprinkled with parsley.

Serving Suggestions: Serve with crushed swede or sweet potatoes, and cabbage.

Storage: Can be refrigerated for 24 hours and reheated until piping hot. The stew by itself can be frozen for later use.

Pork and Butternut Squash Cumberland Pie

Serves: 4 or 5   **Prep:** 25 minutes   **Cook:** 25 minutes
508kcal and 14.1g fat (¼ recipe)
406kcal and 11.3g fat per serving (⅕ recipe)

A savoury base of pork mince with cider, onion, sage and apple is topped with the squash mixture before a delicious crumb-and-cheese coating finishes the pie. Out of season, look for frozen ready-prepared butternut squash.

500g lean pork mince (average fat content 8%)

1 medium onion, finely chopped

1 medium apple, grated

250ml dry cider

1 tsp dried sage

Black pepper

750g potatoes, peeled

1. Place the pork mince in a non-stick saucepan and add the onion. Cook over a medium heat, stirring frequently for about 10 minutes until the pork is browned.

2. Add the apple, cider and sage, and season with black pepper.

3. Cover and allow to simmer for 15 minutes.

4. Preheat oven to 180°C/160°C Fan/GM4.

5. Meanwhile boil or steam the potatoes until tender, and drain.

6. Steam the butternut squash, or cook according to the packet instructions if using frozen or ready-prepared.

¼ serving

NUTRITIONAL ANALYSIS PER PORTION		Protein g	35	Fat g	14.1	Sodium mg	291
		Carbohydrate g	60.2	Of which saturates g	6.1	Salt g	0.7
Kcal	508	Of which sugars g	15.2	Fibre g	7.5	Portion fruit and veg	1½

⅕ serving

NUTRITIONAL ANALYSIS PER PORTION		Protein g	27.9	Fat g	11.3	Sodium mg	232
		Carbohydrate g	48.1	Of which saturates g	4.9	Salt g	0.6
Kcal	406	Of which sugars g	12.1	Fibre g	6.5	Portion fruit and veg	1½

500g butternut squash, peeled and cubed

Grated nutmeg to taste

2 slices (70g) granary bread, made into breadcrumbs

40g Red Leicester cheese, finely grated

7. Mash the squash and potatoes together, adding a little grated nutmeg.

8. Spoon the mince mixture into an ovenproof dish and top with the potato–squash mix.

9. Mix together the breadcrumbs and cheese, and spoon over the potato.

10. Place in the preheated oven and bake for 25 minutes.

11. Serve at once.

Serving Suggestions: Serve with broccoli or green beans.

Storage: Can be frozen or refrigerated for 2 days.

Pork in Dijon Mustard Sauce with Leek Mash

Serves: 2 **Prep:** 10 minutes **Cook:** 15 minutes

500kcal and 12.8g fat per portion

Pork chops need not be fatty, especially if you trim off any visible fat. Pork is a great source of the B vitamin thiamin, which helps release energy from food.

400g potatoes, peeled and quartered

100ml skimmed milk

50g leek, sliced finely

2 tsp rapeseed oil

240g thin lean loin chops, trimmed of all fat

60g (1 small) red onion, finely chopped

100ml dry cider

25g (1 rounded tbsp) Dijon mustard

15g (1 level tbsp) cornflour

Black pepper

1. Boil the potatoes in plenty of unsalted water.
2. Place the milk and sliced leek in a saucepan and gently heat. Allow to simmer for 5 minutes, then turn off the heat and allow to cool.
3. Heat the oil in a non-stick saucepan and gently brown the chops on both sides, then add the onion and fry gently for 5 minutes to soften the onion.
4. Add the cider and mustard to the pan, and cook gently, covered, for 10 minutes to cook the pork through.
5. Remove a little of the cooking liquid and mix with the cornflour. Add back to the pan with the pork and stir until thickened.
6. Drain the cooked potatoes and strain a little of the milk from the leeks into the potato pan. Mash the potatoes until smooth.
7. Stir in the leeks and season with pepper.
8. Spoon the mash onto warmed plates and top with the pork and sauce.

Serving Suggestions: Serve with steamed broccoli, carrots or peas and sweetcorn.

Storage: Not suitable for storage.

NUTRITIONAL ANALYSIS PER PORTION	Protein g	64.9	Fat g	12.8	Sodium g	0.4
	Carbohydrate g	52.7	Of which saturates g	3.2	Salt g	1
Energy kcal 500	Of which sugars g	5.8	Fibre g	3.0	Portion fruit and veg	0

Pork Patties

Serves: 4   **Prep:** 7–8 minutes   **Cook:** 15 minutes
205kcal and 10.9g fat per portion

Pork patties or burgers with an Eastern influence. You can halve the mixture if you are making it for smaller numbers, and the same mixture is used in the Chinese-style Soup with Tiny Pork Balls (page 81).

3 kaffir lime leaves
  (optional)

2 cloves garlic

2 tsp grated fresh
  ginger root

400g lean pork mince
  (<8% fat)

50g fresh
  breadcrumbs

70g spring onions,
  roughly chopped

1 tbsp olive oil

1. Place the kaffir lime leaves, garlic and ginger in a food processor, and blend until finely chopped.

2. Add the pork mince and breadcrumbs, and whiz until combined.

3. Lastly, using the pulse button, add the spring onions so that they remain fairly intact.

4. Using a little flour, divide the mixture into 8 and shape into patties or small burgers.

5. Warm the oil in a non-stick pan and gently fry the patties for about 7–8 minutes each side, until lightly browned.

6. If you prefer you can lightly spray the oil on the patties and grill, turning halfway through cooking.

7. Serve hot.

Serving Suggestions: Serve in a toasted bun with Tomato and Coriander Salsa (page 239).

Storage: Can be kept chilled for 1 day only. Suitable for freezing once cooked.

NUTRITIONAL ANALYSIS PER PORTION		Protein g	21.1	Fat g	10.9	Sodium mg	0.1
Energy kcal	205	Carbohydrate g	5.6	Of which saturates g	3.7	Salt g	0.25
		Of which sugars g	1	Fibre g	0.9	Portion fruit and veg	0

Pork Tenderloin Stuffed with Apple and Cranberry

Serves: 2   **Prep:** 15 minutes   **Cook:** 45 minutes

485kcal and 11.8g fat per portion

This recipe is great for a special occasion, the cranberry and apple making a piquant stuffing.

400g lean pork tenderloin

½ tsp ground allspice

60g (1 small) red onion, finely chopped

150g (1 medium) Cox eating apple, peeled and chopped

50g dried sweetened cranberries, roughly chopped

1. Preheat oven to 180°C/160°C Fan/GM4. Place a large piece of foil on a baking sheet and spray lightly with oil.

2. Place the tenderloin on a chopping board and with a sharp knife slice lengthwise almost through the meat. Open out and spread with the allspice.

3. Mix together the onion, apple and cranberries in a large bowl and stir in the spices.

4. Place the tenderloin on the foil.

5. Spoon the apple and cranberry mixture into the cavity in the pork.

NUTRITIONAL ANALYSIS PER PORTION		Protein g	4939	Fat g	11.8	Sodium g	0.3
		Carbohydrate g	36.3	Of which saturates g	1.5	Salt g	0.75
Energy kcal	485	Of which sugars g	27.1	Fibre g	2.5	Portion fruit and veg	1

50g lean back bacon

15g (1 level tbsp)
cornflour

100ml red wine

6. Wrap the bacon around the outside of the pork to help keep in the mixture. Secure with a cocktail stick or two or string and wrap up the foil.

7. Bake for 35–40 minutes or until the pork juices run clear when tested with a sharp knife.

8. Carefully tip the cooking juices into a saucepan, and keep the pork warm.

9. Place the cornflour in a small bowl and mix in 2 tablespoons of water. Add this to the pan along with the red wine. Bring to the boil, stirring.

10. Serve the pork, cut into thick slices, with the sauce.

Serving Suggestions: Serve with new potatoes and green beans.

Storage: Can be sliced and served cold if any is left over. Not suitable for freezing.

Pork with Lime and Wine Sauce

Serves: 4   **Prep:** 10 minutes   **Cook:** 60 minutes
300kcal and 5.6g fat per serving

A simple casserole with succulent apricots cooked in wine. Choose the leanest pork you can afford. Tenderloin is ideal, or look for ready-diced pork that is less than 5 per cent fat and is stocked in many supermarkets.

500g very lean pork
400g celery
200g dried apricots
4 juniper berries
Zest and juice of
  1 lime
200ml medium or
  sweet white wine
200ml water
1 tbsp cornflour
3 tbsp water

1. Preheat oven to 170°C/150°C Fan/GM3.

2. Cut the pork into small cubes and place in a large casserole dish.

3. Wash the celery and cut into 2- to 3-cm lengths; add to the casserole along with the apricots.

4. Crush the juniper berries with the flat side of a knife to release the flavours.

5. Using a peeler, remove the zest of the lime in strips and add with the juniper to the casserole.

6. Squeeze the lime juice and mix with the wine and water.

7. Pour over the other ingredients, cover and cook in the oven for 40–45 minutes.

8. Remove from the oven, mix the cornflour with the water and a little of the cooking liquor. Pour this over the casserole and stir in. Return to the oven for 15 minutes. Serve hot.

Serving Suggestions: Serve with brown rice or mashed potatoes with green vegetables.

Storage: Can be stored in the fridge for 2–3 days. Also may be frozen.

NUTRITIONAL ANALYSIS PER PORTION		Protein g	29.8	Fat g	5.6	Sodium mg	182
		Carbohydrate g	25.6	Of which saturates g	1.8	Salt g	0.5
Energy kcal	300	Of which sugars g	25.6	Fibre g	5	Portion fruit and veg	2

Pork with Plums and Chinese Spices

Serves: 4   **Prep:** 5 minutes   **Cook:** 30 minutes

265kcal and 6.9g fat per portion

A simple, tasty dish that makes a quick and easy weekday supper. This tastes delicious served with tagliatelle or noodles.

400g pork fillet, cubed

1 tsp Chinese five spice

300g plums

4 small red onions, quartered

20g muscovado sugar

15g (1tbsp) oyster sauce

1 tbsp rapeseed oil

1. **Preheat oven to 200°C/180°C Fan/GM6.**
2. **Place the pork fillet in an ovenproof dish and sprinkle with the spice.**
3. **Quarter and stone the plums, and add to the dish.**
4. **Add the onions and sprinkle over the sugar.**
5. **Drizzle over the oyster sauce and oil, and place, uncovered, in the oven.**
6. **Cook for 25–30 minutes, basting once during cooking.**
7. **Serve hot.**

Serving Suggestions: Serve with noodles and watercress.

Storage: Can be refrigerated for 2 days. Suitable for freezing.

NUTRITIONAL ANALYSIS		Protein g	34.6	Fat g	6.9	Sodium g	0.2
PER PORTION		Carbohydrate g	17.7	Of which saturates g	3	Salt g	–
Energy kcal	265	Of which sugars g	16.4	Fibre g	3.0	Portion fruit and veg	1

Ragu

Serves: 4   **Prep:** 10 minutes   **Cook:** 40–45 minutes
240kcal and 8.7g fat per portion

A good ragu is very versatile, can be frozen and made into lots of other dishes, so even if you are not a keen cook, this one is worth mastering.

500g extra-lean steak mince

160g (1 medium) onion, finely chopped

2 cloves garlic, crushed

½ red pepper, finely chopped

400g can chopped tomatoes

125ml red wine

30g (1 rounded tbsp) sundried tomato paste

1 tbsp chopped basil leaves

Black pepper

1. Place the mince in a large non-stick pan and gently heat, breaking up the meat with a wooden spoon.

2. As the meat starts to brown add the onion, garlic and pepper, and gently fry, stirring frequently until all the onion is soft and the meat browned.

3. Add the canned tomatoes, wine and tomato paste, and bring to the boil, stirring often.

4. Reduce the heat and add the basil and black pepper.

5. Cook for 30–40 minutes, until the sauce is thickened.

Serving Suggestions: For a classic spaghetti bolognaise, serve one portion of the ragu with 50g (dry weight) spaghetti and 10g grated parmesan: 450kcal and 12.5g fat.

Storage: The ragu can be stored in the fridge for 2–3 days, or may be frozen.

NUTRITIONAL ANALYSIS PER PORTION	Protein g	27.9	Fat g	8.7	Sodium g	0.2
	Carbohydrate g	7.1	Of which saturates g	2.8	Salt g	0.5
Energy kcal 240	Of which sugars g	5.7	Fibre g	1.5	Portion fruit and veg	1

Skewered Pork and Mango

Serves: 2   **Prep:** 15 minutes + 20 marianating   **Cook:** 15 minutes
205kcal and 5.4g fat per serving

A simple recipe, great for entertaining, especially if you are barbecuing. Look for
very lean pork, either as frozen diced pork or by asking for pork fillet (tenderloin)
at the butcher's.

250g very lean pork

**Rind and juice of
  1 lime**

**1 small bird's eye chilli
  (optional)**

**100g (1 medium)
  courgette**

150 mango cubes

1. **Cut the pork into cubes about 1.5 cm in size.**
2. **Grate the lime rind finely and place in a bowl, then squeeze in the juice.**
3. **Finely chop the chilli, if using, and add to the bowl.**
4. **Add the pork cubes, stir and cover; then refrigerate and allow to marinate for a minimum of 20 minutes.**
5. **Cut the courgette into slices about 1.5-cm thick.**
6. **Alternately thread mango, pork and courgette onto skewers.**
7. **Grill or barbecue, turning halfway, until the pork is cooked through. This should take about 10–12 minutes depending on the heat of your grill.**
8. **Serve at once.**

Serving Suggestions: Served with 50g (dry weight)
couscous: 288kcal and 4.6g fat per serving.

Storage: This is best eaten at once. Not suitable
for keeping.

NUTRITIONAL ANALYSIS		Protein g	28.2	Fat g	5.4	Sodium mg	90
PER PORTION		Carbohydrate g	11.6	Of which saturates g	1.9	Salt g	0.2
Kcal	205	Of which sugars g	11.0	Fibre g	3.2	Portion fruit and veg	1

Spicy Lamb

Serves: 4   **Prep:** 15 minutes   **Cook:** 90 minutes
302kcal and 13.9g fat per portion

A host of different spices liven up this lamb dish. You can make this in advance as the flavours will improve on keeping. Sainsbury's Be Good to Yourself diced lamb contains less than 3 per cent fat and helps keep the fat content in this dish down.

2 tbsp sunflower or rapeseed oil

200g (1 large) onion, finely chopped

4 cloves garlic, crushed

2 tsp grated fresh ginger root

1 tbsp ground cumin

1 tbsp ground coriander

700g extra-lean lamb, cubed

400g can chopped tomatoes

1 whole green chilli

450ml water (approximately)

1 heaped tbsp garam masala

1 heaped tbsp fresh coriander

1. Preheat oven to 170°C/150°C Fan/GM3.
2. Heat the oil in a large non-stick sauce pan and gently fry the onion, garlic and ginger until softened.
3. Stir in the cumin and ground coriander; adding a little water to prevent sticking if necessary.
4. Add the lamb and tomatoes, the chilli, if using, and enough water just to cover.
5. Cover and place in the preheated oven. Cook for 1 hour, then check to see how tender the meat is, and stir in the garam masala. Return to the oven for another 20–30 minutes until the lamb is cooked through.
6. Serve garnished with the fresh coriander.

Serving Suggestions: Serve with basmati rice, green beans and 1 tbsp of low-fat Raita (see page 247).

Storage: Can be kept in the fridge for 2–3 days and can also be frozen.

NUTRITIONAL ANALYSIS		Protein g	40.7	Fat g	13.9	Sodium g	0.06
PER PORTION		Carbohydrate g	10.5	Of which saturates g	3.2	Salt g	0.2
Energy kcal	302	Of which sugars g	5.8	Fibre g	5.4	Portion fruit and veg	1½

Steak and Mangetout Stir-Fry

Serves: 2   Prep: 10 minutes   Cook: 10 minutes

370kcal and 9.3g fat per portion

Enjoy a piece of steak in this stir-fry. With lots of vegetables and rice you'll be surprised just how far it will go!

100g basmati rice

1 tbsp rapeseed oil

150g lean rump steak, cut into strips

30g (3) spring onions, sliced

200g mangetout, trimmed

80g (about 4–5) baby sweetcorn, sliced

1 head pak choi, chopped

1 tsp grated fresh ginger root

1 tsp finely chopped lemon grass

1 tbsp soy sauce

2 tbsp dry sherry or **Chinese wine**

1. Cook the rice according to the packet instructions.

2. Heat the oil in a non-stick wok and add the steak, stirring frequently until just browned. Remove from the pan and keep warm.

3. Add the spring onions, mangetout and baby sweetcorn with a little water, and quickly cook for 3–4 minutes.

4. Add the steak back to the pan, along with the pak choi, and continue to cook until the pak choi is just wilted.

5. Mix together the ginger, lemon grass, soy sauce and sherry, and pour over the steak. Quickly stir to heat through.

6. Drain the rice and serve immediately with the steak and vegetables.

Tip: Look for bottles of ready-prepared lemon grass.

Storage: Not suitable for storage.

NUTRITIONAL ANALYSIS		Protein g	25.4	Fat g	9.3	Sodium g	0.6
PER PORTION		Carbohydrate g	42.1	Of which saturates g	1.7	Salt g	1.5
Energy kcal	370	Of which sugars g	5.1	Fibre g	6.6	Portion fruit and veg	2

Steak with Sage and Red Wine Sauce

Serves: 2   **Prep:** 10 minutes   **Cook:** 40 minutes

320kcal and 11.9g fat per portion

Tender beef with a herb sauce, which fits within your diet targets too! Buy the leanest steak you can afford, and enjoy a glass of wine while it cooks. A 175ml glass of red wine will provide you with about 119kcal, so don't forget to add to your daily total.

1 tbsp olive oil

2 x 150g lean rump steak

60g (1 small) onion, finely sliced

2 cloves garlic, finely sliced

15g (1 level tbsp) flour

125ml red wine

250ml beef stock

Black pepper

2–3 sage leaves, roughly chopped

1 tbsp chopped fresh parsley to serve

1. Heat the oil in large non-stick pan and lightly brown the steak on both sides. Remove from the heat and keep the steak warm.

2. Add the onion and garlic to the pan, and fry for 5 minutes. Stir in the flour then add the wine and stock.

3. Season with black pepper and the sage leaves, and bring to the boil.

4. Return the steak to the pan, cover and turn the heat right down so that the sauce just bubbles occasionally. Continue cooking, stirring occasionally, for 20–30 minutes until the steak is tender and the sauce is velvety.

5. Serve sprinkled with parsley.

Serving Suggestions: Serve with tagliatelle and a crisp green salad.

Storage: Not suitable for storage.

NUTRITIONAL ANALYSIS PER PORTION		Protein g	33.9	Fat g	11.9	Sodium g	0.3
		Carbohydrate g	10	Of which saturates g	3.4	Salt g	0.8
Energy kcal	320	Of which sugars g	2.2	Fibre g	0.8	Portion fruit and veg	0

Topside with Winter Vegetables

Serves: 4   **Prep:** 15 minutes   **Cook:** 90 minutes
315kcal and 7.8g Fat per portion

An easy winter favourite that uses lean topside or silverside, both cuts of beef that usually come rolled, making them easier for you to handle.

1 tbsp rapeseed oil

600g piece lean
   topside

320g (2 medium)
   onions, quartered

500g carrots,
   washed and cut into
   large chunks

300g turnip, peeled
   and cut into cubes

2 bay leaves

900ml water and
   1 beef stock cube
   or 900ml diluted
   beef stock

15g (1 level tbsp)
   cornflour

1. Preheat oven to 170°C/150°C Fan/GM3.
2. Heat the oil in a large non-stick pan and quickly brown the meat all over. Remove from the heat.
3. Place all the vegetables in the base of a large casserole and put the meat on top.
4. Add the bay leaves and stock, and cover.
5. Place in the oven for 60 minutes, removing and basting the meat with the cooking juices twice.
6. After 1 hour turn up the heat to 200°C/180°C Fan/GM6 and remove the lid. Cook for another 20–30 minutes to allow the meat to brown.
7. Place the vegetables in a warmed serving dish and cut the meat into thick slices.
8. Make a gravy by draining off the cooking juices and mix with 1 tablespoon of cornflour. Bring to the boil to thicken.

Serving Suggestions: Serve with a green vegetable (such as broccoli) and potatoes.

Storage: Any left over can be kept in the fridge for 2 days, and reheated until piping hot. Not suitable for freezing.

NUTRITIONAL ANALYSIS							
PER PORTION	Protein g	37.2	Fat g	7.8	Sodium g	0.4
	Carbohydrate g	26.2	Of which saturates g	2.2	Salt g	1
Energy kcal	315	Of which sugars g	16.8	Fibre g	5.9	Portion fruit and veg	2½

Beef Koftas with Tzatziki

Serves: 2   **Prep:** 15 minutes   **Cook:** 15 minutes

325kcal and 14.3g fat per portion

Make your own beef koftas (meatballs on a kebab stick) using lean beef and Mediterranean vegetables. Served with cool tzatziki you'll feel like you are back on holiday!

250g extra-lean beef
  mince

60g (1 small) onion

1 clove garlic

1 tsp oregano

160g (1) red pepper,
  cubed

125g (1 medium)
  courgette, sliced

Oil spray

For the tzatziki

100g cucumber,
  peeled and grated

150g fat-free Greek
  yogurt

1 clove garlic,
  crushed

1 tbsp finely chopped
  fresh mint

1. Soak 4 wooden skewers in warm water or use 4 metal skewers.

2. Mix together the mince, onion, garlic and oregano in a food processor. Roll into 8 small balls.

3. Thread the meat koftas, pepper and courgette onto the skewers.

4. Lightly spray the vegetables with oil and place the skewers under a hot grill for 10–15 minutes until the meat is cooked through.

5. Make the tzatziki by pressing the cucumber in a sieve to release as much liquid as you can. Discard the liquid.

6. Mix the cucumber with the yogurt, garlic and mint.

7. Serve while the koftas are still hot.

Serving Suggestions: Serve with wholemeal pitta bread: a 60g wholemeal pitta with half the recipe of koftas and tzatziki: 460kcal and 16.g fat.

Storage: The koftas can be kept in the fridge for 1 day, and the tzatziki will keep for 2 days. Not suitable for freezing.

NUTRITIONAL ANALYSIS							
PER PORTION	Protein g	37	Fat g	14.3	Sodium g		Trace
	Carbohydrate g	12.1	Of which saturates g	5.7	Salt g		Trace
Energy kcal	325	Of which sugars g	10.7	Fibre g	2.6	Portion fruit and veg	1½

Fish and Seafood

Bacon-wrapped Pollack
with Baked Cherry Tomatoes

Serves: 1   **Prep:** 5 minutes   **Cook:** 25 minutes
350kcal and 12.3g fat per portion

White fish such as pollack is very low in fat, so you can get away with using bacon, which also imparts a delicious flavour to the fish.

25g (1 rasher)
streaky bacon
150g fillet pollack
1 bay leaf
90g cherry tomatoes

1. **Preheat oven to 190°C/170°C Fan/GM5.**
2. **Wrap the bacon around the fillet and tuck in the bay leaf. Secure with a cocktail stick.**
3. **Place in a small ovenproof dish and add the cherry tomatoes.**
4. **Cook for 20–25 minutes until the fish is cooked through.**

Serving Suggestions: Serve with Crushed New Potatoes with Herbs and Olive Oil (see page 215) and petits pois.

Storage: Not suitable for storage.

NUTRITIONAL ANALYSIS	Protein g		31.3	Fat g	12.3	Sodium g	0.4
PER PORTION	Carbohydrate g		29	Of which saturates g	4.1	Salt g	1
Energy kcal	350	Of which sugars g	4.5	Fibre g	3.5	Portion fruit and veg	1

Trout Fillet with Crushed Peas

Serves: 1   **Prep:** 10 minutes   **Cook:** 15–20 minutes

308kcal and 14.1g Fat per portion

The trout here is kept moist by cooking it 'en papillote' – that is, in a parcel of foil. You could add different vegetables to cook with the trout such as fennel or baby corn.

60g baby asparagus

50g roasted peppers in oil, drained and cut into thin slices

1 tsp chopped fresh dill

150g trout fillet, skin on and any tiny bones removed

20ml lemon juice (about ½ a lemon)

For the peas

100g frozen peas, thawed

1 tbsp chopped fresh mint

1 tsp olive oil

Black pepper

1. Preheat oven to 200°C/180°C Fan/GM°6..

2. Cut a square of foil about 30cm x 30cm.

3. In the centre of the foil place the baby asparagus and cover with the slices of peppers.

4. Sprinkle with the dill then place the trout on top, skin-side up.

5. Squeeze over the lemon juice and scrunch up the foil to cover. Put on a baking sheet and cook for 15 minutes. Then open the foil parcel and return to the oven for 5 minutes to allow the skin to crisp a little.

6. Meanwhile place the peas in a small pan and squash with a potato masher. Add the mint, oil and black pepper, and heat gently till piping hot.

7. When the fish is cooked, slide the fish and vegetables onto a hot serving plate and serve with the crushed peas.

Serving Suggestions: Serve with couscous or new potatoes.

Storage: Not suitable for storage.

NUTRITIONAL ANALYSIS		Protein g	36.4	Fat g	14.1	Sodium g	0.2
PER PORTION		Carbohydrate g	8.8	Of which saturates g	2.6	Salt g	0.5
Energy kcal	308	Of which sugars g	6.2	Fibre g	5.6	Portion fruit and veg	2

Cherry Tomato
and Smoked Haddock Kedgeree

Serves: 2   **Prep:** 20 minutes   **Cook:** 20 minutes

450kcal and 12.8g fat per serving

Add this to your list of brunch recipes as it is a great way to start the day when you haven't got to rush around. It also makes a delicious supper dish; just fork through some peas for a complete meal.

120g smoked haddock or cod fillet

1 tsp olive oil

60g (1 small) onion, finely chopped

18g (1 tbsp) curry paste

150g basmati rice

300ml water

120g cherry tomatoes, halved

5g (1 tsp) low-fat spread

1 hardboiled egg, sliced

1 tbsp chopped fresh coriander

1. Poach the haddock fillet in a little water or cook on Medium in the microwave.
2. Meanwhile heat the oil in a large non-stick saucepan and gently fry the onion for 3–4 minutes.
3. Stir in the curry paste and 1 tablespoon of water to prevent sticking if you need to.
4. Rinse the (dry) basmati rice and add to the pan along with the water.
5. Bring to the boil and then reduce the heat, cover and cook gently until the rice is tender.
6. Meanwhile cook the tomatoes in the low-fat spread in a non-stick pan, until they are soft and pulpy.
7. To serve, flake the cooked fish and carefully stir through the rice along with the cooked tomatoes. Top with the egg and fresh coriander.

Serving Suggestions: Fork through a serving of peas per person (80g x 2) for a main meal.

Storage: The kedgeree is best served fresh and hot.

NUTRITIONAL ANALYSIS PER PORTION		Protein g	23	Fat g	12.8	Sodium mg	775
		Carbohydrate g	61.8	Of which saturates g	1.7	Salt g	1.9
Energy kcal	450	Of which sugars g	3.9	Fibre g	1	Portion fruit and veg	1

Italian Tuna with Black Olives and Tomatoes

Serves: 2   **Prep:** 5–10 minutes   **Cook:** 15–20 minutes
420kcal and 12.2g fat per portion

Crisp-coated tuna with a sweet tomato sauce. You'll not feel like you're on a diet with this recipe.

2 slices granary bread

1 tsp dried Italian herbs

2 x 150g tuna steaks

10g (2 tsp) pesto

200g canned tomatoes

25g black olives in brine, sliced

4–5 basil leaves, torn

1 tsp sugar

1 tbsp balsamic vinegar

1. **Preheat oven to 190°C/170°C Fan/GM5.**
2. **Make breadcrumbs with the granary bread, stir in the Italian herbs and place in a shallow bowl.**
3. **Spread the tuna with the pesto very sparingly.**
4. **Press the tuna into the breadcrumbs and coat each piece.**
5. **Bake the tuna for 15–20 minutes.**
6. **Meanwhile place the tomatoes, olives and basil in a pan, and simmer gently. Add the sugar and vinegar, and continue to cook for 10 minutes.**
7. **Serve the tuna on a bed of the sauce.**

Serving Suggestions: Serve with boiled new potatoes and steamed mangetout.

Storage: Not suitable for storage.

NUTRITIONAL ANALYSIS		Protein g	53.4	Fat g	12.2	Sodium g	0.7
PER PORTION		Carbohydrate g	25	Of which saturates g	2.5	Salt g	1.75
Energy kcal	420	Of which sugars g	6.8	Fibre g	3.3	Portion fruit and veg	1

Lemony Salmon with Thyme Couscous and Onion Salad

Serves: 1   **Prep:** 10 minutes   **Cook:** 10 minutes

410kcal and 15.3g fat per portion

A vitamin-C rich salad whose citrus flavours are a great foil to the oily salmon.

100g fillet salmon

Juice of 1 lemon

50g (dry weight) couscous

80ml boiling water

60g (1 small) red onion, finely sliced

90g (1) medium ripe plum tomato, sliced

1 tbsp balsamic glaze

1 tbsp chopped fresh thyme

30g wild rocket

1. Place the salmon on a heatproof plate and spoon over half the lemon juice.
2. Cook the salmon on Medium in the microwave for 4–5 minutes, or steam over a pan until the flesh flakes and is opaque throughout.
3. Meanwhile pour boiling water onto the couscous and allow it to swell. Leave, covered, for 5 minutes.
4. Make the salad by laying out the onion on a serving plate and topping with the slices of tomato. Drizzle over the balsamic glaze.
5. When the couscous is ready, fork through the thyme leaves and the remaining lemon juice.
6. Add the couscous to the serving plate and top with the rocket and salmon. Serve at once.

Serving Suggestions: Try this using another fish, such as fresh tuna or grilled sardines.

Storage: Not suitable for storage.

NUTRITIONAL ANALYSIS PER PORTION		Protein g	20.6	Fat g	15.3	Sodium g	trace
		Carbohydrate g	47.3	Of which saturates g	4	Salt g	Trace
Energy kcal	410	Of which sugars g	10.8	Fibre g	1.8	Portion fruit and veg	1½

Monkfish and Prawn Kebabs

Serves: 2   Prep: 10 minutes + 30 marianating   Cook: 10–12 minutes
202kcal and 7.7g fat per portion

For a special summer barbecue these kebabs are the business. Any chunky, firm fish will do just as well as the monkfish if you don't feel like pushing the boat out.

1 tbsp fish sauce

2 cloves garlic, crushed

2 tsp grated fresh ginger root

1 tbsp chopped fresh coriander leaves

1 tbsp olive oil

2 tbsp fresh lemon juice

150g monkfish, cut into large cubes

100g raw peeled tiger prawns

100g (1 medium) courgette, cut into 1cm slices

160g baby yellow or orange peppers, cut in half lengthwise

2 stalks lemon grass, each cut into 4

1. Make the marinade by blitzing the fish sauce, garlic, ginger, coriander, olive oil and lemon juice together in a blender.

2. Pour the marinade over the monkfish and prawns, and leave to marinate for 30 minutes.

3. Meanwhile soak 4 wooden skewers.

4. When you are ready to barbecue, thread the prawns, courgette, fish, peppers and lemon grass onto the skewers.

5. Barbecue for 10–12 minutes or place under a hot grill until the fish is cooked though.

6. Serve at once.

Serving Suggestions: Serve with Coconut Rice (page 214): 1 portion Coconut Rice with 2 skewers is 386kcal and 12.2g fat.

Storage: Not suitable for storage.

NUTRITIONAL ANALYSIS PER PORTION		Protein g	26.6	Fat g	7.7	Sodium g	0.9
		Carbohydrate g	6.5	Of which saturates g	1.1	Salt g	2.25
Energy kcal	202	Of which sugars g	5.6	Fibre g	1.8	Portion fruit and veg	1

Pickled Herring with Beetroot Slaw

Serves: 1   **Prep:** 10 minutes

360kcal and 13.6g fat per portion

A crunchy and tangy salad is an ideal companion to pickled herring. Don't forget that you should be aiming for at least one portion of oily fish a week.

80g (1 small) raw
  beetroot

70g (1 small) Cox
  apple

Juice of ½ a lemon

1 tbsp chives, snipped

1 tsp olive oil

30g (a handful)
  rocket

90g pickled (rollmop)
  herring

1. **Peel and grate the beetroot (you may want to wear vinyl gloves to prevent your hands from staining) and place in a bowl.**

2. **Grate in the apple and mix with the lemon juice, chives and oil.**

3. **Place the rocket on a salad plate and top with the beetroot salad.**

4. **Serve the pickled herring on the side.**

Serving Suggestions: Just add some fresh wholemeal bread to complete your meal: 1 medium slice adds 70kcal and 0.8g fat.

Storage: The beetroot slaw will keep in the fridge for 24 hours. Not suitable for freezing.

NUTRITIONAL ANALYSIS	Protein g	18.4	Fat g	13.6	Sodium g	0.9
PER PORTION	Carbohydrate g	41	Of which saturates g	0.6	Salt g	2.25
Energy kcal	360	Of which sugars g	22.6	Fibre g	3.1	Portion fruit and veg	2

Plaice and Parma Ham Rolls with Roasted Vegetables

Serves: 2　Prep: 10 minutes　Cook: 30 minutes

365kcal and 12.2g fat per portion

Plaice is often overlooked as a white fish, but its delicate flavour is enhanced here by the addition of Parma ham.

2 x 175g plaice fillets

56g (4 slices) Parma ham

125g (1 medium) courgette, finely sliced

100g (half) fennel bulb, finely sliced

120g (about 8) baby plum tomatoes

1 tbsp olive oil

Few basil leaves

Juice of 1 lemon

250g baby new potatoes

1. Preheat oven to 200°C/180°C Fan/GM6.
2. Remove any visible bones from the fish, and cut each fillet in half lengthwise. Place a piece of ham on each fillet and roll up each piece, securing with a cocktail stick.
3. Place the vegetables in a bowl and pour in the oil. Mix well before tipping into an ovenproof dish. Place the rolls of fish on top and tuck in the basil leaves. Pour over the lemon juice.
4. Bake for 30 minutes until the fish flakes easily and looks opaque. After 20 minutes, put the new potatoes on to boil.
5. Serve with the boiled potatoes.

Serving Suggestions: Add a green salad or mangetout.

Storage: Not suitable for storage.

NUTRITIONAL ANALYSIS PER PORTION		Protein g	40.8	Fat g	12.2	Sodium g	0.8
		Carbohydrate g	22.5	Of which saturates g	2.5	Salt g	2
Energy kcal	365	Of which sugars g	4.5	Fibre g	1.7	Portion fruit and veg	1½

Polenta-crusted Cod
with Tarragon Sauce

Serves: 2   **Prep:** 5 minutes   **Cook:** 25 minutes

210kcal and 5.1g fat per portion

Try this different take on breaded cod. You can choose another white fish, if you prefer.

25g polenta (dry meal)

1 egg white, beaten

2 x 125g pieces cod fillet

100g fromage frais

Zest of ½ a lemon and 1 tbsp lemon juice

1 tsp chopped fresh tarragon

1. Preheat oven to 190°C/170°C Fan/GM5 and lightly spray a baking sheet with oil.
2. Place the polenta in a small bowl.
3. Place the egg white in a shallow bowl and dip the cod to cover it.
4. Now dip the cod in the polenta and place on the baking sheet.
5. Bake for 15–30 minutes depending on the thickness of the cod, until the cod flakes.
6. Meanwhile mix the fromage frais with the zest, lemon juice and the fresh tarragon.
7. Serve the hot cod with the tarragon sauce.

Serving Suggestions: Serve with new potatoes and peas.

Storage: The cod is not suitable for storage. The dip may be kept in the fridge for up to 2 days.

NUTRITIONAL ANALYSIS PER PORTION		Protein g	28.4	Fat g	5.1	Sodium g	0.1
		Carbohydrate g	13.3	Of which saturates g	2.9	Salt g	0.2
Energy kcal	210	Of which sugars g	2.2	Fibre g	0	Portion fruit and veg	0

Prawns with Sweet Potato and Lime

Serves: 2　　**Prep:** 10 minutes　　**Cook:** 20 minutes

305kcal and 9g Fat per portion

This recipe uses harissa, which is a North African mixture of spices and chilli in oil. You only need a tiny quantity of this fiery pepper paste and if you can't buy it or prefer to use something else then a curry paste would be a good alternative.

1 tbsp olive oil

160g (1 medium) onion, finely chopped

1 clove garlic, crushed

250g sweet potato, peeled and cut into approximately 1-cm cubes

1 teaspoon harissa paste or curry paste

200ml water

Pinch of ground cardamom

250g cooked peeled prawns

Juice of 1 lime

1. Heat the oil in a non-stick pan and gently fry the onion and garlic.
2. Add the sweet potato and the harissa or curry paste.
3. Stir in the water and the cardamom, and bring to the boil.
4. Reduce the heat, cover and simmer for 15 minutes until the sweet potato is just tender.
5. Stir in the prawns and the lime juice, and heat through until hot.
6. Serve at once.

Serving Suggestions: Serve with 50g (dry weight) basmati rice and steamed spinach.

Storage: This can be stored for 1 day in the fridge. Reheat until piping hot. Not suitable for freezing.

NUTRITIONAL ANALYSIS PER PORTION		Protein g	26.1	Fat g	9	Sodium g	0.7
		Carbohydrate g	31.7	Of which saturates g	1.6	Salt g	1.8
Energy kcal	305	Of which sugars g	10.7	Fibre g	5.3	Portion fruit and veg	½

Scallop and Prawn Chow Mein

Serves: 4   **Prep:** 10–15 minutes   **Cook:** 10 minutes

422kcal and 10.2g fat per portion

If you have a special occasion and are worried about eating out, this is the answer. It serves 4 people, is very quick to make and contains delicious ingredients. Look for packs of frozen scallops, which are much cheaper than fresh ones. Just thaw and dry on kitchen paper.

250g egg noodles

2 tbsp rapeseed oil

50g (5) spring onions, roughly sliced

100g red pepper, sliced

100g green pepper, sliced

10g grated fresh ginger root

2 garlic cloves, crushed

135g frozen scallops, defrosted

200g cooked peeled king prawns

300g fresh beansprouts

100g sweet chilli stir-fry sauce, e.g. Waitrose

1. Cook the egg noodles according to the packet instructions, drain and keep warm.

2. Heat 1 tablespoon of the oil in a non-stick wok or large pan, and stir-fry the onions and peppers, then stir in the ginger and garlic.

3. In a separate pan heat the other spoon of oil and gently fry the scallops for 2–3 minutes, then add the prawns and fry for another 2–3 minutes, stirring often.

4. Meanwhile add the beansprouts to the wok and stir-fry for another minute or so to heat through.

5. Stir the chilli sauce and drained noodles into the wok and lastly add the hot shellfish and stir through.

6. Serve at once.

Serving Suggestions: Replace the noodles with rice. A portion of the stir-fry with 50g per person (dry weight) basmati rice provides 400kcal and 9.5g fat.

Storage: Not suitable for storage.

NUTRITIONAL ANALYSIS PER PORTION		Protein g	25.7	Fat g	10.2	Sodium mg	0.7
		Carbohydrate g	57.4	Of which saturates g	1.4	Salt g	1.8
Energy kcal	422	Of which sugars g	12.6	Fibre g	5.4	Portion fruit and veg	1½

Seabass with Lemon Grass and Baby Corn

Serves: 2   **Prep:** 5 minutes   **Cook:** 20 minutes

190kcal and 4.4g fat per portion

An Eastern approach to seabass fillets, but made very easy by using a foil pouch to keep the fish moist.

80g (half) red pepper, very finely sliced

120g (about 8) baby corn, halved lengthwise

4 spring onions, chopped

1 tsp very lazy chilli or 1 bird's eye chilli, finely chopped

1 tsp chopped lemon grass

2 x 150g fillets sea-bass with skin left on

1. Preheat oven to 190°C/170°C Fan/GM5.
2. Cut 2 pieces of foil large enough to wrap around each fillet.
3. Place the red pepper on the foil and add the corn and spring onions.
4. Spread the chilli and lemon grass on the flesh of each bass fillet.
5. Place the fillet, skin-side up, on the vegetables and make a parcel with the foil.
6. Put each fish parcel on a baking sheet and bake for 12–15 minutes.
7. Open the parcel and return to the oven for 5 or so minutes to allow the skin to crisp up a little.
8. Serve at once.

Serving Suggestions: Serve with basmati rice and stir-fried vegetables.

Storage: Not suitable for storage.

NUTRITIONAL ANALYSIS PER PORTION		Protein g	31.8	Fat g	4.4	Sodium g	Trace
		Carbohydrate g	5.7	Of which saturates g	0.7	Salt g	Trace
Energy kcal	190	Of which sugars g	5.1	Fibre g	2.6	Portion fruit and veg	1

Seafood Paella

Serves: 4   **Prep:** 15 minutes   **Cook:** 25–30 minutes
416kcal and 6g fat per portion

There are as many versions of paella as there are Spanish restaurants, some including chicken as well as fish. This one uses white fish and shellfish cooked in fish stock for a full seafood flavour.

1 tbsp olive oil
60g (1 small) onion, finely chopped
1 tsp ground turmeric
1 red pepper, diced
250g short-grain rice
50ml dry white wine
2 tsp chopped dill
500ml fish stock
200g white fish fillets (haddock, pollack, hoki, cod or coley), cut into chunks
250g mussels, cleaned
80g sweetcorn
250g cooked king prawns, tail on

1. In a large non-stick shallow pan, heat the oil and cook the onion with the turmeric and pepper for 5 minutes until they are softened.
2. Stir in the rice, wine, dill and fish stock, and bring to the boil. Simmer for 10 minutes, stirring frequently.
3. Add the white fish, mussels and sweetcorn, and cook until the fish is starting to flake. Discard any mussels that do not open. Add more stock as required to prevent sticking.
4. Stir in the prawns and heat through until piping hot.
5. Serve at once.

Serving Suggestions: Quarter some lemons to use for additional piquancy.

Storage: Not suitable for storage.

NUTRITIONAL ANALYSIS PER PORTION	Protein g	34.4	Fat g	6	Sodium g	1.4
	Carbohydrate g	54.1	Of which saturates g	0.8	Salt g	3.5
Energy kcal 416	Of which sugars g	7.2	Fibre g	1.3	Portion fruit and veg	½

Simple Cod Bake

Serves: 2   **Prep:** 5 minutes   **Cook:** 25 minutes

260kcal and 8.7g fat per portion

Any white fish will do for this recipe, so choose one that is sustainably sourced.

200g tomatoes, sliced

1 tsp snipped chives

200g white fish fillets, skinned (cod, hoki, haddock, pollack)

Black pepper (optional)

70g (2 slices) granary bread, made into breadcrumbs.

40g mature cheddar, grated

1. **Preheat oven to 200°C/180°C Fan/GM6.**
2. **Cover the base of an ovenproof dish with the tomato slices and sprinkle over the chives.**
3. **Add the fish fillets and grind over a little pepper if desired.**
4. **Mix the breadcrumbs with the cheese and spread over the fish.**
5. **Bake for 20–25 minutes until the fish is cooked and the top crispy and golden brown.**
6. **Serve at once.**

Serving Suggestions: Serve with sugar snaps or mangetout.

Storage: Not suitable for storage.

NUTRITIONAL ANALYSIS		Protein g	26.5	Fat g	8.7	Sodium g	0.4
PER PORTION		Carbohydrate g	19.8	Of which saturates g	4.7	Salt g	1
Energy kcal	260	Of which sugars g	4.1	Fibre g	2.5	Portion fruit and veg	1

Smoked Haddock Fish Cakes

Serves: 4   **Prep:** 25 minutes   **Cook:** 20 minutes
306kcal and 9.5g fat per portion

Nothing beats home-made fish cakes and you can choose the fish that suits your budget and palate. This uses smoked haddock with a little peppadew to give it a kick. You could use an unsmoked fish if you prefer.

400g undyed smoked
   haddock
400g floury
   potatoes, such as
   Maris Piper
40g (1 rounded tbsp)
   reduced-fat crème
   fraîche
25g olive spread
15g chopped fresh
   parsley

1. Place the fish in a pan of cold water and bring to simmering point. Cook for 3–4 minutes or until the fish just starts to flake. Remove from the water; drain and remove the skin.
2. Meawhile boil the potatoes until just soft.
3. Drain and mash the potatoes with the crème fraîche and olive spread until fluffy.
4. Stir in the fish, parsley and, if using, the chopped peppadew peppers. Season with black pepper.
5. Allow to cool for 15 minutes before shaping into 8 patties, using a little flour to prevent sticking if necessary.

NUTRITIONAL ANALYSIS PER PORTION		Protein g	25.3	Fat g	9.5	Sodium g	0.6
		Carbohydrate g	31.8	Of which saturates g	3.7	Salt g	1.5
Energy kcal	306	Of which sugars g	4.3	Fibre g	3.0	Portion fruit and veg	0

30g peppadew
  peppers (optional)
Black pepper
1 medium egg, beaten
108g (3 slices)
  wholemeal bread,
  made into
  breadcrumbs

6. Meanwhile preheat oven to 200°C/180°C Fan/GM6, and lightly spray a baking sheet with oil.
7. Place the beaten egg and breadcrumbs in 2 separate shallow bowls.
8. Dip the fish cakes in egg to cover, then in the breadcrumbs to coat before placing on the baking sheet. Bake for 15–20 minutes until they are golden brown.
9. Serve hot.

Serving Suggestions: Serve with a crisp salad and a glass of white wine.

Storage: May be stored in the fridge for 1 day prior to cooking, or 1 day after cooking. May also be frozen once cooked.

Special Fish Pie

Serves: 4   **Prep:** 20 minutes   **Cook:** 30 minutes

400kcal and 8.2g fat per portion

Fish in white sauce is a classic, and this version contains a seafood medley of mussels, prawns and calamari. Served with petits pois, it is a complete meal all the family will enjoy.

350g skinned white fish fillets, such as cod, coley, haddock or pollack

500ml semi-skimmed milk

150g (1 medium) leek, cut into rings

2 bay leaves

Few peppercorns

800g floury potatoes

25g olive spread

30g white flour

10g chopped parsley

1. Place the fish in a large flat pan and pour over 400ml of the milk.
2. Add the leek, bay leaves and peppercorns, and heat very gently to poach the fish.
3. When the fish flakes easily, lift it out with a draining spoon and place in a large, shallow ovenproof dish. Strain the milk to remove the leeks, bay leaves and peppercorns. Save the leeks.
4. Meanwhile peel and boil the potatoes until they are just tender.
5. Preheat oven to 180°C/160°C Fan/GM4.
6. Melt the spread in a non-stick pan and stir in the flour to make a roux. Gradually stir in the reserved milk and bring to the boil, stirring all the time to make a smooth sauce, then, off the heat, add the parsley.

NUTRITIONAL ANALYSIS		Protein g	34.9	Fat g	8.2	Sodium g	0.5
PER PORTION		Carbohydrate g	45.9	Of which saturates g	3.1	Salt g	1.25
Energy kcal	400	Of which sugars g	10.6	Fibre g	3.8	Portion fruit and veg	0

250g pack seafood medley or 250g cooked peeled prawns

50ml skimmed milk

7. **Scatter the saved leeks and the seafood medley or prawns over the fish, and pour over the parsley sauce.**

8. **Mash the potatoes with the skimmed milk until creamy, then spoon onto the fish pie.**

9. **Bake for 30 minutes until the potato is lightly browned.**

10. **Serve at once.**

Serving Suggestions: Serve with petits pois or sweetcorn.

Storage: Can be made and stored before baking for 24 hours if the fish is completely fresh. Can be frozen once cooked.

Sundried Tomato-topped Seafood Bake

Serves: 2   **Prep:** 5 minutes   **Cook:** 20–25 minutes

180kcal and 6.5g fat per serving

A simple fish recipe that can use any white fish. Try basa, which is a cheaper alternative to over-fished cod and haddock.

250g white fish fillets, such as basa

100g cooked peeled prawns

50g sundried tomatoes in oil, drained and chopped

1 tbsp chopped fresh parsley

Juice and grated rind of 1 lemon

1. **Preheat oven to 180°C/160°C Fan/GM4.**
2. **Place the fish and prawns in an ovenproof dish.**
3. **Top with the tomatoes and parsley.**
4. **Sprinkle over the grated lemon rind and juice.**
5. **Cover and place in the oven for 15–20 minutes. Halfway through cooking time, remove to baste with the cooking liquor.**

Serving Suggestions: Serve with new potatoes and vegetables such as mangetout with baby sweetcorn. Served with 175g boiled new potatoes: 323kcal and 7.4g fat.

Storage: This is not suitable for storage.

NUTRITIONAL ANALYSIS PER PORTION						
	Protein g	30	Fat g	6.5	Sodium mg	471
	Carbohydrate g	0.3	Of which saturates g	0.2	Salt g	1.1
Energy kcal	180	Of which sugars g	0.2	Fibre g	0.2	Portion fruit and veg	0

Baked Plaice with Warm Lentil Salad

Serves: 2   **Prep:** 15 minutes   **Cook:** 30 minutes

217kcal and 3.8g fat per portion

Plaice has a delicate flavour and is cooked very simply here. The earthy flavours of the raw beetroot and whole lentils make a great accompaniment as well as providing fibre and B vitamins.

60g green lentils

1 tsp olive oil

60g (1 small) red onion, very finely chopped

1 clove garlic

20ml fresh lemon juice

60g (1 small) raw beetroot

2 plaice fillets (130g)

Black pepper

1 tbsp flat leaf parsley, chopped

1. Boil the lentils until just tender but still whole. Drain.
2. Preheat oven to 190°C/170°C Fan/GM5.
3. Heat the oil in a non-stick pan, and fry the onion and garlic until lightly browned. Remove from the heat and stir in the lemon juice.
4. Peel and roughly grate the beetroot, and stir into the warm onion mixture.
5. Meanwhile dry the plaice with kitchen paper and cut in half lengthwise. Place the fish on a lightly greased baking sheet and season with a little pepper. Bake for 10–12 minutes until the fish is opaque.
6. Mix the lentils and parsley with the beetroot mixture and spoon onto 2 serving plates.
7. Serve with the plaice fillets on top.

Serving Suggestions: A few new potatoes will complete your meal.

Storage: The lentil salad can be kept in the fridge for up to 3 days. Not suitable for freezing.

NUTRITIONAL ANALYSIS		Protein g	28.2	Fat g	3.8	Sodium g	0.1
PER PORTION		Carbohydrate g	17.1	Of which saturates g	0.5	Salt g	0.2
Energy kcal	217	Of which sugars g	3.9	Fibre g	3.8	Portion fruit and veg	1

Tandoori Fish with Spicy Okra

Serves: 2   **Prep:** 10 minutes   **Cook:** 25 minutes

400kcal and 11g fat per portion

A spicy fish served with okra in a yogurt sauce. Use coley or another inexpensive white fish, as the spices tend to mask any delicate fish flavour.

300g coley fillets or similar white fish, skinned

150g carton fat-free Greek yogurt

35g (1 rounded tbsp) tandoori curry paste

Juice of 1 lime

1 tbsp olive oil

200g okra, trimmed and halved lengthwise

1 tsp grated fresh ginger root

2 cloves garlic

1 small green chilli, finely chopped

80g basmati rice

1 tbsp fresh coriander leaves

1. Preheat oven to 200°C/180°C Fan/GM6.

2. Wipe the fish with kitchen paper to dry.

3. Take 2 level tablespoons of the yogurt and mix with the curry paste and half the lime juice.

4. Spread this mixture over the fish and put to one side while you prepare the okra.

5. Heat the oil in a non-stick pan and fry the okra for 5 minutes, stirring frequently to prevent sticking. Add the ginger, garlic and chilli and 50–100ml water to prevent sticking. Cover and cook gently for 10–15 minutes or until the okra is tender.

6. Cook the rice according to the packet instructions.

7. Meanwhile place the fish on a non-stick baking sheet in the preheated oven. Bake for 15 minutes or until the fish flakes easily.

8. While the fish is cooking, add the remaining lime juice, the coriander and the rest of the yogurt to the okra. Stir and warm through but do not allow to boil.

9. Serve the rice on a warmed plate then add the okra and top with the fish.

Storage: The fish can be marinated overnight in the fridge. Not suitable for freezing.

NUTRITIONAL ANALYSIS			Protein g	41.1	Fat g	11	Sodium g	0.4
PER PORTION			Carbohydrate g	35.1	Of which saturates g	1.2	Salt g	1.0
Energy kcal		400	Of which sugars g	4.9	Fibre g	2.5	Portion fruit and veg	1

Mediterranean Fish in Filo Parcels

Serves: 1   **Prep:** 5 minutes   **Cook:** 15 minutes

270kcal and 13.4g fat per portion

Look for grilled Mediterranean vegetables in olive oil, known as Escalavida. Sardines are a wonderful source of omega-3 fatty acids as well as zinc and iron, and because the bones are also eaten they provide calcium, too.

1 tsp olive oil or oil-mister

24g (2 average sheets) filo pastry

50g Escalavida (grilled Mediterranean vegetables in olive oil), drained

80g sardines canned in brine, drained

1 clove garlic, crushed

1 tbsp fresh lemon juice

1. Preheat oven to 200°C/180°C Fan/GM6.
2. Lightly spray or brush one sheet of filo with oil and place on a baking sheet. Spray the second sheet and lay on top of the other at a 90-degree angle to the first.
3. If the grilled vegetables are large, cut into strips.
4. Place the sardines in the centre of the pastry and top with the grilled vegetables, then sprinkle over the garlic and lemon juice.
5. Fold in one end of the pastry and roll over the parcel. Tuck in the ends and roll to enclose the contents completely. Lightly spray with oil and bake for 12–15 minutes.
6. Serve hot or at room temperature.

Serving Suggestions: Serve with a crisp green salad.

Storage: Not suitable for storage.

NUTRITIONAL ANALYSIS		Protein g	20.3	Fat g	13.4	Sodium g	0.7
PER PORTION		Carbohydrate g	16.3	Of which saturates g	0.8	Salt g	1.75
Energy kcal	270	Of which sugars g	4.7	Fibre g	0.3	Portion fruit and veg	0

Vegetarian Dishes

Chipotle Lentils

Serves: 4   **Prep:** 10 minutes   **Cook:** 40 minutes
295kcal and 11.2g fat per portion

Chipotle paste has a lovely hot, smoky flavour, which tastes wonderful when mixed with lentils.

250g green or brown lentils

1 tbsp sunflower oil

160g (1 medium) onion, finely chopped

2 cloves garlic, crushed

400ml water

10g (2 tsp) chipotle chilli paste

150g half-fat crème fraîche

2 tbsp chopped coriander

1. Place the lentils in a pan and cover with water. Bring to the boil and boil for 10 minutes. Drain.
2. Heat the oil in a non-stick pan and gently brown the onion and garlic.
3. Add the partially cooked lentils, water and chipotle paste, and bring to the boil. Cover and simmer until the lentils are soft, about 30 minutes. Add more water as required to keep the mixture moist but not swamped.
4. Mix the crème fraîche and coriander, and stir in just before serving.

Serving Suggestions: Serve with basmati rice or a tortilla wrap with Tomato and Red Onion Salad (see page 137).

Storage: May be kept refrigerated for up to 3 days. Also suitable for freezing.

NUTRITIONAL ANALYSIS PER PORTION		Protein g	15.9	Fat g	11.2	Sodium g	Trace
		Carbohydrate g	31.9	Of which saturates g	5.3	Salt g	Trace
Energy kcal	295	Of which sugars g	4.1	Fibre g	6.1	Portion fruit and veg	1

Tricolour Risotto

Serves: 4   **Prep:** 15 minutes   **Cook:** 45 minutes
450kcal and 11.3g fat per portion

This looks so pretty – deep purple beetroot, orange squash and the vibrant green peas. If you like to 'eat a rainbow' for your 5 a day, here are 3 in one course.

300g butternut squash, cubed

300g raw beetroot, quartered

1 tbsp plus 1 tsp olive oil

150g shallots, sliced

50ml vermouth or dry white wine

300g risotto rice

700–800ml vegetable stock

250g petits pois, defrosted

100g parmesan, grated

1. **Preheat oven to 200°C/180°C Fan/GM6.**
2. **Place the squash and beetroot in a mixing bowl, and pour over the tablespoon of olive oil, then mix around to cover the vegetables with the oil. Tip into a baking tray and roast for 35–45 minutes or until the vegetables are tender.**
3. **About 20 minutes into the cooking time, heat the teaspoon of oil in a large non-stick pan and fry the shallots until they are lightly browned.**
4. **Stir in the vermouth or wine and rice, and stir around to coat the rice in the oil.**
5. **Add about half the stock and bring the risotto slowly to the boil. Simmer, adding more stock and stirring until the rice is soft, around 25 minutes.**
6. **In the last 5 minutes, add the petits pois.**
7. **When the risotto is completely cooked serve on warmed plates with the roasted vegetables, topped with the parmesan.**

Serving Suggestions: Omit the squash and beetroot and add 250g mushrooms, or some edamame (soya) beans.

Storage: Not suitable for storage.

NUTRITIONAL ANALYSIS		Protein g	16.9	Fat g	11.3	Sodium g	0.2
PER PORTION		Carbohydrate g	74	Of which saturates g	4.6	Salt g	0.5
Energy kcal	450	Of which sugars g	13.5	Fibre g	7.2	Portion fruit and veg	3

Galettes with Spinach, Mushroom and Goat's Cheese

Serves: 1   **Prep:** 20 minutes   **Cook:** 15 minutes
320kcal and 12.5g fat per portion

Galettes are savoury pancakes made from buckwheat flour or sarasin. This recipe makes 8 galettes and enough filling for 2.

75g buckwheat or wholemeal flour
75g plain flour
2 medium eggs
300ml skimmed milk
Oil-mister

For the filling
1 tsp olive oil
100g chestnut mushrooms, sliced
30g baby spinach leaves
50g soft mild goat's cheese (10% fat)
85g (1 medium) ripe tomato, sliced
Balsamic glaze

1. Make the galettes by mixing together the flours, eggs and milk in a blender or processor to achieve a smooth pouring batter. Heat a small non-stick frying pan and when hot spray lightly with oil.
2. Pour enough batter to coat the bottom of the pan thinly when swirled around.
3. Cook until the edges are curling then turn over and cook the other side.
4. Lift out of the pan and keep warm.
5. Repeat with the remaining mixture to make 8 galettes in all.
6. For the filling for 2 galettes, heat the oil in a non-stick pan and sweat the mushrooms for 5 minutes over a low heat. Stir and continue to cook gently until the mushrooms have 'collapsed'.
7. Add the spinach leaves and cover.
8. When the spinach has wilted stir in the soft cheese and remove from the heat.
9. To serve, spread and roll up two galettes with the spinach/cheese mixture. Serve with the tomato slices drizzled with balsamic glaze.

Storage: The cooked plain galettes will keep in the fridge for 2 days, or can be frozen.

NUTRITIONAL ANALYSIS PER PORTION	Protein g	19.7	Fat g	12.5	Sodium g	Unknown
	Carbohydrate g	31.9	Of which saturates g	1.8	Salt g	Unknown
Energy kcal 320	Of which sugars g	8.7	Fibre g	4	Portion fruit and veg	2

Lentil and Spinach Dhal with Cardamom

Serves: 4   **Prep:** 10 minutes   **Cook:** 30 minutes
210kcal and 4.5g fat per portion

A simple and inexpensive meal that is low in fat and high in fibre. It also provides plenty of iron. All you need is some rice and a spoonful of raita as accompaniments.

1 tbsp rapeseed oil

160g (1 medium) onion, finely chopped

2 cloves garlic, crushed

10g (2 tsp) grated fresh ginger root

1 tbsp ground cumin

1 tbsp ground turmeric

200g split red lentils

8 cardamom pods, split

500ml water

170g frozen spinach, thawed and drained

30g chopped fresh coriander

1. Heat the oil in a large non-stick pan and gently fry the onion and garlic for a few minutes to brown them lightly.

2. Add the ginger, cumin and turmeric, and a little water to prevent sticking, and cook for 1 minute.

3. Stir in the lentils and cardamon pods along with the water.

4. Bring to the boil, stir and simmer for 20 minutes, adding more water if necessary to allow the lentils to swell and become soft.

5. When the lentils are nearly tender, add the spinach and heat through.

6. Before serving stir in the coriander.

Serving Suggestions: Served with 40g (dry weight) basmati rice per person and a quarter (75g) of the Raita recipe (see page 247): 375kcal and 4.7g fat.

Storage: Suitable for freezing. Can also be stored in an airtight container in the fridge for 2–3 days.

NUTRITIONAL ANALYSIS PER PORTION		Protein g	13.3	Fat g	4.5	Sodium g	Trace
		Carbohydrate g	28.9	Of which saturates g	0.4	Salt g	Trace
Energy kcal	210	Of which sugars g	3.4	Fibre g	3	Portion fruit and veg	1½

Mushroom and Feta Filo Pouches

Serves: 2   **Prep:** 15 minutes   **Cook:** 15–20 minutes

235kcal and 9.8g fat per serving

These little filo pouches look fiddly but are in fact easy to make. You can use a range of different types of fillings, substituting peppers, courgettes or tomatoes for the mushrooms. Use an oil-mister to minimize fat.

125g button
  mushrooms
100g feta cheese
1 small red onion
Black pepper
Sprig of rosemary,
  finely chopped
4 tsp olive oil – or use
  an oil-mister
180g (4 large sheets)
  filo pastry

1. Preheat oven to 190°C/170°C Fan/GM5.
2. Wipe the mushrooms and cut into quarters. Place in a bowl.
3. Cut the feta into small cubes and add to the bowl.
4. Finely slice the onion and stir into the mushroom mixture.
5. Season with black pepper and the rosemary. (Feta is salty, so don't add salt.)
6. Lightly brush or spray the filo pastry with oil, and fold in half.
7. Spoon one-quarter of the mixture into the centre of the pastry and draw up the corners to make a pouch.
8. Transfer to a baking sheet and spray lightly all over with oil.
9. Make 3 more pouches in this way.
10. Bake for 15–20 minutes until golden.
11. Serve warm (2 pouches per person).

Serving Suggestions: Serve with salad leaves and a piece of chunky bread.

Storage: These are best eaten fresh.

NUTRITIONAL ANALYSIS PER PORTION		Protein g	9.4	Fat g	9.8	Sodium mg	586
		Carbohydrate g	27.1	Saturates	4.2	Salt equivalent g	1.5
Energy kcal	235	Of which sugars	3.9	Fibre g	0.5	Portion fruit and veg	½

Mushroom Stroganoff with Rice

Serves: 2   Prep: 5 minutes   Cook: 15 minutes

430kcal and 13.4g fat per portion

This light vegetarian stroganoff uses reduced-fat sour cream, though for an even lighter version you could use buttermilk or fat-free yogurt. Choose whichever mushrooms you like – combining varieties provides more flavour.

1 tbsp olive oil

160g (1 medium) onion, finely sliced

300g mushrooms, sliced

1 tsp chopped fresh thyme

100g basmati rice

15g (1 level tbsp) cornflour

150ml dry white wine

150ml reduced-fat sour cream

1 tbsp chopped fresh parsley

1. Heat the oil in a non-stick pan and gently fry the onion for 2–3 minutes.

2. Add the prepared mushrooms and thyme, cover and allow them to sweat over a low heat for 5–10 minutes, stirring occasionally, until they are soft.

3. Meanwhile cook the rice according to the packet instructions.

4. Mix the cornflour with the wine and stir in to the mushroom mix, allowing it to thicken.

5. Add the sour cream and parsley, heat gently and serve with the rice.

Serving Suggestions: Add some peas or broccoli spears.

Storage: Not suitable for storage.

NUTRITIONAL ANALYSIS		Protein g	11.3	Fat g	13.4	Sodium g	Trace
PER PORTION		Carbohydrate g	53.4	Of which saturates g	5.1	Salt g	Trace
Energy kcal	430	Of which sugars g	6.7	Fibre g	2.8	Portion fruit and veg	2

Pepperonata with Baked Eggs

Serves: 2   **Prep:** 10 minutes   **Cook:** 40 minutes
250kcal and 13.4g fat per portion

Pepperonata is a Mediterranean pepper stew, and in this version eggs are oven-baked with the pepperonata.

1 tbsp olive oil	1. **Preheat oven to 190°C/170°C Fan/GM5.**
160g (1 medium) onion, sliced	2. **Heat the oil in a non-stick pan and gently fry the onion and garlic until lightly browned.**
2 cloves garlic, crushed	3. **Stir in the peppers and tomatoes, and cook for 15 minutes, stirring occasionally.**
480g (3 medium) peppers, any colour, sliced	4. **Tip the mixture into a lightly greased shallow dish and make two 'nests' for the eggs.**
340g (4 medium) tomatoes, skinned and cut into quarters	5. **Break an egg into each hollow and place in the oven for 15–20 minutes until the eggs are set.**
2 large eggs	6. **Serve at once.**

Serving Suggestions: Serve with some crusty bread.

Storage: Not suitable for storage.

NUTRITIONAL ANALYSIS	Protein g	11.9	Fat g	13.4	Sodium g	Trace
PER PORTION	Carbohydrate g	20	Of which saturates g	2.9	Salt g	Trace
Energy kcal	250	Of which sugars g	18	Fibre g	6.4	Portion fruit and veg	2

Stuffed Butternut Squash

Serves: 4   Prep: 15 minutes   Cook: 70–80 minutes
290kcal and 13.6g fat per portion

Butternut squash is readily available and is a great source of beta-carotene, the plant form of vitamin A.

1 butternut squash
(about 850g)
1 tsp olive oil
160g (1 medium) red
onion, finely
chopped
150g celery, finely
chopped
72g (2 slices) granary
bread
64g (4 tbsp)
sunflower seeds
1 tbsp fresh thyme
leaves
1 tbsp chopped fresh
parsley
50g stilton cheese

1. **Preheat oven to 200°C/180°C Fan/GM6.**
2. **Cut the squash in half and scoop out the seeds.**
3. **Place the halves on a baking sheet and bake for 45 minutes or until the flesh is tender.**
4. **Meanwhile sweat the onion and celery in the olive oil in a non-stick pan.**
5. **Place the bread and half the sunflower seeds in a food processor and blend.**
6. **Add the herbs and pulse to mix together.**
7. **When the squash is cooked, combine the breadcrumb mixture with the onion and celery, and crumble in the stilton.**
8. **Spoon the crumble into the cavity of the squash, and sprinkle over the remaining seeds.**
9. **Return to the oven for 20 minutes or until the mixture is golden and the cheese melted.**
10. **Cut each half into half again and serve.**

Serving Suggestions: Add some cherry tomatoes, or a crisp salad.

Storage: Not suitable for storage.

NUTRITIONAL ANALYSIS							
PER PORTION	Protein g	11.5	Fat g	13.6	Sodium g	0.2	
	Carbohydrate g	30.1	Of which saturates g	3.7	Salt g	0.5	
Energy kcal	290	Of which sugars g	12.2	Fibre g	6	Portion fruit and veg	1½

Courgette and Celery Filo Pie

Serves: 4   **Prep:** 20 minutes   **Cook:** 30–40 minutes

216kcal and 12.3g fat per portion

Filo pastry is a great boon to dieters as it is low in fat and can be used to make interesting parcels containing succulent food. Minimize fat by using an oil spray or mister.

180g (2 medium) courgettes

250g celery

1 tbsp olive oil

4 spring onions, roughly chopped

20g fresh parsley, finely chopped

10g fresh sage, finely chopped

Black pepper

1. Preheat oven to 200°C/180°C Fan/GM6.
2. Wipe and slice the courgettes finely. Wash and drain the celery and slice finely.
3. Gently heat the olive oil in a large non-stick pan and add the courgettes and celery. Sweat these over a low heat for about 10 minutes, stirring often to prevent sticking.
4. Remove from the heat and add the spring onions, parsley and sage. Grind over black pepper and mix well. Allow to cool slightly.
5. Lightly spray a 20-cm round pie tin with oil.

NUTRITIONAL ANALYSIS		Protein g	8.8	Fat g	12.3	Sodium g	0.2
PER PORTION		Carbohydrate g	18	Of which saturates g	5.5	Salt g	0.6
Energy kcal	216	Of which sugars g	5	Fibre g	2.3	Portion fruit and veg	1½

Oil-mister

100g filo pastry
  sheets

250g ricotta cheese

6. Using the oil-mister, lightly spray 4 sheets of the
   filo pastry and place one by one in the pie tin so
   that they overlap and cover the edge of the tin.

7. Stir the ricotta cheese into the vegetable
   mixture and spoon into the pie tin.

8. Fold over the filo edges partly to cover
   the mixture.

9. Spray the remaining filo sheets with the oil and
   use to cover the top of the pie, scrunching up the
   pastry for a crumpled effect on top.

10. Bake for 35–40 minutes until the pie is
    golden brown.

11. Remove from the oven and allow to cool slightly
    before serving.

Serving Suggestions: Serve with sliced tomatoes and
crusty bread.

Storage: The pie will keep in the fridge for 2–3 days.

Three Bean Curry

Serves: 4   **Prep:** 10 minutes   **Cook:** 40 minutes
200kcal and 4.5g fat per portion

Low in fat and high in fibre, this bean curry is great for the dieter. You can use any beans you like, soaking and boiling dry ones if you prefer. This recipe uses canned beans for speed. Look out for varieties which are canned in water rather than with added salt and sugar.

1 tsp olive oil

160g (1 medium) onion, finely chopped

2 cloves garlic, crushed

10g (2 tsp) grated ginger

2 tsp ground turmeric

2 tsp ground cumin

1–2 birdeye chillies

400g can butterbeans

400g can kidney beans

400g can cannellini beans

200g can chopped tomatoes

1 tbsp garam masala

1 tbsp coriander leaves, chopped

1. Heat the oil in a non-stick pan and fry the onion, garlic, and ginger until softened, adding a little water to prevent sticking if necessary.
2. Stir in the turmeric, cumin, chilli and bayleaves.
3. Tip in all the beans, and the tomatoes along with 200ml of water and bring to the boil, stirring occasionally.
4. Cover and reduce the heat and allow to simmer for 15 minutes, stirring every now and then and checking that the curry has sufficient water.
5. Cook for another 20 minutes, then taste the curry.
6. Add the garam masala to taste and finally the chopped coriander.
7. Serve hot.

Serving Suggestions: Served with one portion Coconut Rice and Raita: 407kcal and 9.1g fat.

Storage: Will keep, and improve if kept in the fridge overnight. Will keep up to 3 days. Best not frozen.

NUTRITIONAL ANALYSIS PER PORTION		Protein g	12.6	Fat g	4.5	Sodium g	0.3
		Carbohydrate g	27.7	Of which saturates g	0.5	Salt g	0.8
Energy kcal	200	Of which sugars g	6.3	Fibre g	8.6	Portion fruit and veg	2

Sides

Apricot and Ginger Rice

Serves: 2   **Prep:** 5 minutes   **Cook:** 20 minutes
200kcal and 3.7g Fat per portion

Simple, but delicious, basmati rice is low in GI so will keep hunger at bay.

60g (1 small) onion, finely chopped

2 tsp olive oil

1 tsp grated fresh ginger root

60g basmati rice, rinsed

50g dried apricots, chopped

160–200ml vegetable stock

1 tbsp chopped fresh parsley

1. **In a non-stick pan, fry the onion in the olive oil until just soft.**
2. **Add the ginger, rice and apricots.**
3. **Pour in 160ml of the stock and bring to the boil.**
4. **Cover and simmer, checking every few minutes and adding more stock if required.**
5. **Serve sprinkled with parsley.**

Serving Suggestions: Serve with stir-fries, stews or grilled meats.

Storage: Not suitable for storage.

NUTRITIONAL ANALYSIS		Protein g	3.9	Fat g	3.7	Sodium g	0.2
PER PORTION		Carbohydrate g	38.1	Of which saturates g	0.4	Salt g	0.5
Energy kcal	200	Of which sugars g	13.4	Fibre g	2.5	Portion fruit and veg	½

Watercress and Orange Salad

Serves: 2   **Prep:** 5 minutes

115kcal and 0.6g fat per portion

A fresh citrussy salad which tastes great with grilled meat or poultry.

30g watercress

20g lamb's lettuce

200g (1 large) orange, peeled and cut into segments

160g (1 medium) pear, finely sliced

Half recipe for Apple and Mint Dressing (page 238)

1. **Wash the watercress and remove any thick stalks.**
2. **Place the cress and lamb's lettuce on a serving dish and arrange the orange and pear slices on top.**
3. **Spoon over the apple and mint dressing.**
4. **Serve at once.**

Serving Suggestions: Adding 20g pecan nuts or walnuts, chopped finely gives 180kcal and 7.4g fat.

Storage: Not suitable for storage.

NUTRITIONAL ANALYSIS		Protein g	2	Fat g	0.6	Sodium g	4.1
PER PORTION		Carbohydrate g	25.2	Of which saturates g	0.6	Salt g	Trace
Energy kcal	115	Of which sugars g	25	Fibre g	Trace	Portion fruit and veg	2

Braised Red Cabbage

Serves: 4   **Prep:** 10 minutes   **Cook:** 60–90 minutes
85kcal and 0.5g fat per portion

This classic favourite makes an excellent accompaniment to pork dishes, or any type of roast. It cooks alongside other dishes in the oven.

**500g red cabbage,
roughly chopped
160g (1) red onion,
finely sliced
200g (1 medium)
cooking apple,
peeled, cored and
roughly chopped
½ tsp ground
cinnamon
12g (2 heaped tsp)
demerara sugar
25g (1 tbsp) sultanas
15ml (1 tbsp) wine
vinegar**

1. **Preheat oven to 170°C/150°C Fan/GM4.**
2. **Place all the ingredients in an ovenproof casserole, cover and place in the oven.**
3. **After 1 hour check that the cabbage is not drying out, adding a little water if it is. Stir and return to the oven.**
4. **Continue to cook until all the ingredients are tender.**

Serving Suggestions: Serve with a baked potato and grilled low-fat sausages.

Storage: Suitable for freezing and for storage in the fridge for 2–3 days.

NUTRITIONAL ANALYSIS	Protein g		2	Fat g		0.5	Sodium g		Trace
PER PORTION	Carbohydrate g		17.6	Of which saturates g		Trace	Salt g		Trace
Energy kcal	85	Of which sugars g		16.5	Fibre g		4.4	Portion fruit and veg	2

Citrus Couscous

Serves: 4   **Prep:** 5 minutes   **Cook:** 10 minutes
248kcal and 0.2g fat per portion

This is an extremely easy accompaniment, which adds zing to grilled fish or chicken. This makes enough for 4 good portions, but nutrition information for 6 portions is provided, too.

200g couscous
1 lime
1 large orange
100g sultanas
225ml boiling water

1. Place the couscous in a large bowl.
2. Finely grate the rinds from the lime and orange, and add to the couscous along with the sultanas.
3. Squeeze the juice from the lime and orange, and stir into the couscous.
4. Lastly stir in the boiling water and leave for 10 minutes.
5. Using a fork, fluff up the couscous.
6. Serve warm or cold.

Serving Suggestions: Try with grilled chicken or fish or cold with 80g cooked green beans and 1 tbsp (15g) of pinenuts as a delicious salad: 375kcal and 11.5g fat.

Storage: Will keep in the fridge for 2 days, though the amount of vitamin C from the citrus fruit will decrease over time.

Serves 4

NUTRITIONAL ANALYSIS PER PORTION		Protein g	6.9	Fat g	0.2	Sodium mg	Trace
		Carbohydrate g	55.8	Of which saturates g	0	Salt g	Trace
Energy kcal	248	Of which sugars g	20.2	Fibre g	1.5	Portion fruit and veg	1

Serves 6

NUTRITIONAL ANALYSIS PER PORTION		Protein g	4.6	Fat g	0.1	Sodium mg	Trace
		Carbohydrate g	37.2	Of which saturates g	0	Salt g	Trace
Energy kcal	165	Of which sugars g	13.5	Fibre g	1	Portion fruit and veg	1

Coconut Rice

Serves: 4   **Prep:** 5 minutes   **Cook:** 15 minutes
170 kcal and 4.5g fat per portion

Coconut is high in fat, but big on taste, so you can get a lot of flavour when using small amounts. Coconut sold in a block called creamed coconut is easy to measure out.

160g white basmati rice
350ml boiling water
25g creamed coconut, roughly chopped

Optional spices:
Cardamom pods
Cinnamon sticks
Bay leaves

1. **Rinse the rice and drain well.**
2. **Place in a saucepan and pour over the boiling water, the coconut and the spices.**
3. **Bring to the boil, stir, cover and turn off the heat. The rice will cook through by itself within about 10–12 minutes.**
4. **Fork through before serving, removing any large spices.**

Serving suggestions: Serve with curries, or casseroles.

Storage: Not suitable for storage.

NUTRITIONAL ANALYSIS PER PORTION:	Protein g	3.7	Fat g	4.5	Sodium g	0
	Carbohydrate g	29	Of which saturates g	3.7	Salt g	0
Energy kcal 170	Of which sugars g	0.4	Fibre g	0	Portion fruit and veg	0

Crushed New Potatoes with Herbs and Olive Oil

Serves: 1   **Prep:** 5 minutes   **Cook:** 15 minutes

135kcal and 3.5g fat per portion

This recipe, though very simple, has been created so that you can keep a handle on your fat and calorie intake while enjoying fully flavoured food.

150g baby new
potatoes (about 6)

1 tsp olive oil

Black pepper

1 tsp chopped fresh
herbs, e.g. mint,
parsley, chervil,
coriander

1. Scrub the new potatoes.
2. Boil or steam them whole until they are just tender – about 12–15 minutes.
3. Drain and press with a potato masher to crush lightly.
4. Carefully drizzle over the oil and pepper, and sprinkle with the fresh herbs.

Serving Suggestions: Great with grilled chicken or meat, and tastes lovely with stews, too.

Storage: Not suitable for storing.

NUTRITIONAL ANALYSIS		Protein g	2.1	Fat g	3.5	Sodium g	Trace
PER PORTION		Carbohydrate g	23.2	Of which saturates g	0.6	Salt g	Trace
Energy kcal	135	Of which sugars g	1.6	Fibre g	1.6	Portion fruit and veg	0

Greek Peas with Leek and Mint

Serves: 4   **Prep:** 5 minutes   **Cook:** 10 minutes

95kcal and 4.4g fat per portion

Deliciously simple, this vegetable mixture is full of vitamin C and fibre and an ideal accompaniment to plain grilled meat.

2 tsp olive oil

150g leeks

50ml water

1 tbsp chopped fresh
  mint

150g soya beans

150g petits pois

1. **Heat the olive oil in a large non-stick pan and gently fry the leeks for 5 minutes.**

2. **Add the water and mint, and allow to bubble for a minute or two before adding the soya beans and peas.**

3. **Boil for 5 minutes until all the vegetables are cooked through and hot.**

4. **Serve at once.**

Serving Suggestions: Serve with the Marinated Lamb with Crushed Potatoes (page 152).

Storage: Not suitable for storage.

NUTRITIONAL ANALYSIS	Protein g	7.3	Fat g	4.4	Sodium g	Trace
PER PORTION	Carbohydrate g	6.7	Of which saturates g	0.7	Salt g	Trace
Energy kcal 95	Of which sugars g	1.9	Fibre g	5.8	Portion fruit and veg	1½

Leek and Mustard Mash

Serves: 2   **Prep:** 5 minutes   **Cook:** 20 minutes

185kcal and 1.5g fat per portion

An easy low-fat recipe that is an ideal accompaniment to stews or grills alike.

400g potatoes, e.g.
  King Edward, peeled
  and quartered
100ml skimmed milk
80g leek, finely sliced
15g (heaped tsp)
  wholegrain
  mustard
Black pepper

1. Boil the potatoes in unsalted water until tender, about 15–20 minutes.
2. Place the milk in a saucepan along with the leek and bring to simmering point slowly. Simmer for 5 minutes. Remove from the heat.
3. When the potatoes have cooked, drain them well and return to the pan.
4. Drain the leek from the milk and use the milk to mash with potatoes.
5. When the potatoes are light and fluffy stir in the mustard and black pepper. Finally, add the leeks.
6. Serve at once.

Serving Suggestions: Try this without the mustard, but with 60g strongly flavoured reduced-fat cheddar: 260kcal and 5.4g fat.

Storage: Not suitable for storage.

NUTRITIONAL ANALYSIS		Protein g	7.1	Fat g	1.5	Sodium g	0.1
PER PORTION		Carbohydrate g	38	Of which saturates g	0.1	Salt g	0.2
Energy kcal	185	Of which sugars g	4.6	Fibre g	3.8	Portion fruit and veg	½

Okra with Tomatoes

Serves: 2 **Prep:** 10 minutes **Cook:** 15 minutes

128kcal and 3.7g fat per portion

This can be served as a side dish with grilled chicken, meat or fish along with some tasty basmati rice.

1 tsp olive oil

2 cloves garlic, crushed

250g (1 large) red onion, sliced

300g okra, topped and tailed and cut into 1-cm pieces

320g (2 large) ripe tomatoes, roughly chopped

Juice of 1 lime

60–90ml (4–6 tbsp) water

1 tbsp chopped parsley or coriander

1. Heat the oil in a non-stick pan and gently fry the garlic and onion until softened.
2. Add the okra and tomatoes, and cook over a low heat, stirring occasionally, for 5 minutes.
3. Stir in the lime juice and half the water.
4. Gently simmer, adding more water, as required, until the okra is tender, about 10–15 minutes.
5. Serve at once with chopped parsley or coriander.

Serving Suggestions: One portion served with 50g (dry weight) basmati rice and 16g (1 tbsp) toasted pinenuts: 415kcal and 15.5g fat.

Storage: Store in an airtight container for 2 days in the fridge. Not suitable for freezing.

NUTRITIONAL ANALYSIS PER PORTION		Protein g	6.8	Fat g	3.7	Sodium mg	Trace
		Carbohydrate g	18	Of which saturates g	1.4	Salt g	Trace
Energy kcal	128	Of which sugars g	14.5	Fibre g	9.1	Portion fruit and veg	3

Polenta with Parmesan and Shallots

Serves: 2 **Prep:** 5 minutes **Cook:** 10 minutes

165kcal and 4.8g fat per portion

Fed up with potatoes or rice? Quick-cook polenta makes a great change, and this version is flavoured with parmesan and shallots.

1 tsp olive oil

60g shallots, finely chopped

250ml water

60g quick-cook polenta

20g parmesan, finely grated

1. Heat the oil in a small non-stick pan and cook the shallots until lightly browned.
2. Measure the water into a saucepan and bring to the boil, then add the polenta and stir while cooking until thickened, about 5 minutes.
3. Stir in the cooked shallots and parmesan, and serve immediately.

Serving Suggestions: Serve with grilled meat or the Ratatouille (page 221).

Storage: If you pour the hot polenta into a baking tin, you can chill and serve it in slices, either grilled or oven-baked.

NUTRITIONAL ANALYSIS PER PORTION		Protein g	5.9	Fat g	4.8	Sodium g	0.1
		Carbohydrate g	24.4	Of which saturates g	2.3	Salt g	0.2
Energy kcal	165	Of which sugars g	1.1	Fibre g	0.4	Portion fruit and veg	0

Potatoes with Mustard Seeds and Spinach

Serves: 2 or 3   **Prep:** 5 minutes   **Cook:** 15–20 minutes

220kcal and 8.3g fat per ½ recipe; 146kcal and 5.6g fat per ⅓ recipe

A typical Indian dish that is so easy to make yourself – without the usual high-fat content. If you prefer to use fresh spinach, cook it separately in a large pan, then drain, press and add instead of the defrosted spinach.

1 tbsp sunflower or rapeseed oil

1 tbsp mustard seeds

1 tsp ground turmeric

400g potatoes, cut into small cubes

200ml boiling water

Pinch salt

200g frozen spinach, defrosted

1. **Heat the oil in a large non-stick pan and add the mustard seeds. Heat gently to allow them to sizzle before adding the turmeric and chopped potatoes.**

2. **Pour over the water and add salt. Cover and simmer for 10–15 minutes until the potatoes are almost tender.**

3. **Stir in the defrosted spinach and heat through.**

4. **Serve warm or hot.**

Serving Suggestions: Delicious served with the Lentil and Spinach Dhal with Cardamon (page 201).

Storage: Will store in the fridge for 2 days. Not suitable for freezing.

Serves 2

NUTRITIONAL ANALYSIS PER PORTION		Protein g	8.9	Fat g	8.3	Sodium g	0.4
		Carbohydrate g	34.4	Of which saturates g	0.9	Salt g	1.0
Energy kcal	220	Of which sugars g	2.1	Fibre g	6.7	Portion fruit and veg	1

Serves 3

NUTRITIONAL ANALYSIS PER PORTION		Protein g	6	Fat g	5.6	Sodium g	0.3
		Carbohydrate g	23	Of which saturates g	0.6	Salt g	0.7
Energy kcal	146	Of which sugars g	1.4	Fibre g	4.4	Portion fruit and veg	1

Ratatouille

Serves: 4 or 6 **Prep:** 15 minutes **Cook:** 45 minutes

85kcal and 1.2g fat per ¼ recipe; 64kcal and 0.8g fat per ⅙ recipe

This recipe comes from the 'bung it in and leave it' school of cookery. A very simple Mediterranean vegetable stew high in vitamins and minerals, which has no added fat and tastes great with chicken or fish.

680g bottle crushed tomatoes

medium red onion, peeled and sliced

200g courgettes, trimmed and sliced into 1-cm pieces

200g (1 small) aubergine, diced

3 cloves garlic, crushed

200g peppers, any colour (you can use ready-sliced frozen)

8–10 basil leaves, torn

1 tsp dried or fresh oregano

1. Pour the crushed tomatoes into a large saucepan and add the onion, courgettes, aubergine and garlic. If you are using fresh peppers, add them with the other vegetables.

2. Add the herbs and bring to the boil. Either cook gently on the hob for 45 minutes or place in a preheated oven at 180°C/160°C Fan/GM4 for about 1 hour.

3. If you are using frozen peppers, add these halfway through cooking to prevent them becoming too soggy.

4. When the vegetables are tender, remove from the heat.

5. Serve warm or at room temperature.

Serving Suggestions: Served with 40g white rice and 50g reduced-fat cheddar: 375kcal and 9.3g fat.

Storage: Can be kept for 2–3 days in the fridge. Can be frozen.

Serves 4

NUTRITIONAL ANALYSIS PER PORTION	Protein g	2.5	Fat g	1.2	Sodium g	Trace
	Carbohydrate g	16.1	Of which saturates g	0.3	Salt g	Trace
Energy kcal 85	Of which sugars g	14.8	Fibre g	3.5	Portion fruit and veg	3

Sweet Potato and Swede Mash

Serves: 2 **Prep:** 5–8 minutes **Cook:** 15–20 minutes
142kcal and 1.3g fat per portion

Very rich in carotenes (the plant version of vitamin A) and low in GI, this simple mash is a great accompaniment for stews.

250g swede, peeled and cut into dice

250g sweet potato, peeled and cut into dice

Grating of fresh nutmeg

Black pepper

1. Place the swede in a saucepan of boiling water and bring back to the boil. Cover and simmer for 5 minutes before adding the sweet potato.

2. Continue cooking until both vegetables are tender.

3. Drain and mash until smooth, adding the nutmeg and pepper.

4. Serve at once.

Serving Suggestions: Serve with any of the delicious casserole recipes in this book.

Storage: Not suitable for storage.

NUTRITIONAL ANALYSIS	Protein g	2.4	Fat g	1.3	Sodium g	Trace
PER PORTION	Carbohydrate g	30.2	Of which saturates g	0.5	Salt g	Trace
Energy kcal	142	Of which sugars g	12.6	Fibre g	5.4	Portion fruit and veg	2

Warm Potato Salad with Herbs

Serves: 2   **Prep:** 5 minutes   **Cook:** 20 minutes

120kcal and 3.8g fat per portion

A perfect accompaniment for barbecued meat or fish, these potatoes are coated with dressing while hot and allowed to soak up the flavours.

250g new potatoes, scrubbed

2 tsp olive oil

1 tbsp white wine vinegar

1 level tsp wholegrain mustard

1 tbsp snipped fresh chives

1 tbsp chopped fresh parsley

1. **Cut any large potatoes into halves and cook in boiling water until just tender.**

2. **Meanwhile prepare the dressing by whisking together all the remaining ingredients in a large bowl.**

3. **When the potatoes are cooked, drain and then stir into the dressing to coat the potatoes.**

4. **Leave to cool a little before serving.**

Serving Suggestions: Delicious with grilled meat or fish.

Storage: Best served within a couple of hours of preparation.

NUTRITIONAL ANALYSIS		Protein g	2.2	Fat g	3.8	Sodium g	Trace
PER PORTION		Carbohydrate g	19.5	Of which saturates g	0.6	Salt g	Trace
Energy kcal	120	Of which sugars g	1.5	Fibre g	0.3	Portion fruit and veg	0

Boulangère Potatoes

Serves: 4   **Prep:** 5 minutes   **Cook:** 45 minutes

150kcal and 3.4g fat per portion

Boulangère potatoes are cooked in the oven in vegetable stock, usually with onions. If you crave gratin Dauphinois on your diet, these at least are oven-baked and low-fat!

2 tsp olive oil

160g (1 medium) onion, finely chopped

500g floury potatoes, such as Maris Piper or King Edward

2 bay leaves

600ml vegetable stock

1. Preheat oven to 200°C/180°C Fan/GM6.
2. Place the oil in a non-stick pan and gently fry the onion until lightly browned. Add a little water to prevent sticking if necessary.
3. Peel the potatoes and slice thinly.
4. Arrange the potatoes in a shallow ovenproof dish in layers, adding the bay leaves and onion along the way.
5. Pour over enough stock just to cover the potatoes and place in the oven.
6. Bake for 45 minutes, checking occasionally to ensure the fluid hasn't all dried up – add more if this is the case.
7. When the potatoes are tender, serve.

Serving Suggestions: Great with stews, grilled poultry, meat or fish.

Storage: Not suitable for storage.

NUTRITIONAL ANALYSIS		Protein g	3.4	Fat g	3.4	Sodium g	1.90.3
PER PORTION		Carbohydrate g	26.7	Of which saturates g	0.4	Salt g	0.8
Energy kcal	150	Of which sugars g	3.2	Fibre g	1.9	Portion fruit and veg	0

Pasta

Baked Rigatoni with Celery, Ham and Cider

Serves: 2 **Prep:** 10 minutes **Cook:** 15 minutes

500kcal and 7.6g fat per portion

A sweet cider sauce provides a tasty contrast to the ham. Reduced-fat cheese is sprinkled on top before finishing in the oven.

180g rigatoni pasta

200ml dry cider

100g (2 sticks) celery, finely sliced

15g (1 level tbsp) cornflour

10g (1 heaped tsp) wholegrain mustard

50g lean ham, roughly chopped

60g reduced-fat cheddar

1. Cook the pasta according to the packet instructions, then drain and keep warm.

2. Place the cider and celery in a saucepan, and simmer to cook the celery.

3. When the celery is softened, about 5 minutes, mix the cornflour with 1 tablespoon of water and stir into the saucepan.

4. Stir in the mustard and ham, and add the cooked pasta.

5. Pour into an ovenproof dish and sprinkle over the cheese.

6. Place under a preheated grill until the cheese is bubbling.

Serving Suggestions: Serve with Watercress and Orange Salad (page 211).

Storage: Can be stored for 24 hours after you take it out of the oven (but before you pop it under the grill). To reheat, place in a preheated oven and bake for 20 minutes.

NUTRITIONAL ANALYSIS PER PORTION	Protein g	26.8	Fat g	7.6	Sodium g	0.6
	Carbohydrate g	75.8	Of which saturates g	3.7	Salt g	1.5
Energy kcal 500	Of which sugars g	6.4	Fibre g	3.3	Portion fruit and veg	½

Tripoline with Lemon Mushrooms

Serves: 1 **Prep:** 7 minutes **Cook:** 12 minutes
400kcal and 8g fat per portion

Quark is a low-fat soft cheese that is ideal for cooking. In this pasta sauce it provides a creamy base for the lemony mushrooms.

2 tsp garlic-infused oil or olive oil with
1 small clove crushed garlic
100g chestnut mushrooms
Grated zest of 1 lemon
Black pepper
75g tripoline or tagliatelle
100g Quark
50ml water

1. Heat the oil in a non-stick saucepan and sweat the mushrooms for 5 minutes, stirring frequently.
2. Add the lemon zest and black pepper, and continue to cook, covered, for 5 minutes over a low heat.
3. Meanwhile cook the pasta according to the packet instructions, then drain.
4. Off the heat add the Quark to the cooked mushrooms and stir in up to 50ml of hot water to make the sauce a pouring consistency.
5. Combine the pasta and sauce, and serve at once.

Serving Suggestions: Serve with a salad made from baby plum tomatoes and finely sliced red onions, with balsamic glaze.

Storage: Not suitable for storage.

NUTRITIONAL ANALYSIS		Protein g	25.7	Fat g	8	Sodium g	Trace
PER PORTION		Carbohydrate g	60	Of which saturates g	1.1	Salt g	Trace
Energy kcal	400	Of which sugars g	6.9	Fibre g	3.8	Portion fruit and veg	1

Fusilli with Red Pepper and Olive Sauce

Serves: 1   **Prep:** 5 minutes   **Cook:** 15 minutes

465kcal and 12.4g fat per portion

A chunky pasta sauce that is rich in vitamin C and also provides 2 of your 5 a day!
If you prefer a smooth sauce, blend it before serving.

1 tsp olive oil

160g (1 medium) red
pepper, diced

60g (1 small) red
onion, finely
chopped

200g can chopped
tomatoes

10g (1 rounded tsp)
sundried tomato
paste

1 tbsp chopped fresh
basil

25g black olives,
pitted and sliced

Black pepper

75g fusilli

1. Heat the oil in a non-stick saucepan and gently
   fry the pepper and onion until softened.
2. Add the chopped tomatoes and bring to the boil.
3. Reduce the heat and stir in the tomato paste,
   basil, black olives and black pepper.
4. Simmer for 15–20 minutes until the sauce is
   thickened and the flavours are developed.
5. Meanwhile cook the fusilli according to the
   packet instructions.
6. Combine the drained fusilli with the sauce.

Serving Suggestions: Serve with a crisp green salad,
or wilt some spinach and stir into the sauce just
before serving.

Storage: The sauce will keep in the fridge for 2–3 days
in an airtight container. It is also suitable for freezing.

NUTRITIONAL ANALYSIS		Protein g	13.1	Fat g	12.4	Sodium g	0.7
PER PORTION		Carbohydrate g	80.6	Of which saturates g	1.5	Salt g	1.75
Energy kcal	465	Of which sugars g	23.4	Fibre g	8.2	Portion fruit and veg	2

Pasta Sauce with Artichokes and Peppers

Serves: 4   **Prep:** 10 minutes   **Cook:** 25 minutes
106kcal and 6.9g fat per portion

An easy pasta sauce that you can also use to accompany grilled meat or fish. Make sure you drain the artichokes well to remove the oil. If you are not keen on artichokes, try marinated roasted peppers instead (these tend to be lower in fat, too).

1 tbsp olive oil

160g (1 medium) onion, finely chopped

1 clove garlic, crushed

150g marinated artichokes in oil, drained

400g can chopped tomatoes

50g peppadew peppers, roughly chopped (optional)

1 tbsp chopped parsley

Black pepper

1. Heat the oil in a non-stick saucepan and gently fry the onion and garlic until softened.
2. Roughly chop the drained artichokes and add to the pan along with the tomatoes.
3. Add the chopped peppers and parsley.
4. Stir well and bring to simmering point, then reduce the heat. Allow to simmer for 20 minutes until the sauce has thickened and the vegetables are soft.
5. Grind in plenty of black pepper.
6. If you like a chunky sauce serve like this, or if you prefer a smooth sauce, blend to your preferred consistency.

Serving Suggestions: Served with 75g (dry weight) pasta: 374kcal and 8.1g fat.

Storage: The sauce can be stored in the fridge for 2–3 days. It also freezes well.

NUTRITIONAL ANALYSIS			Protein g	2.1	Fat g	6.9	Sodium g	0.3
PER PORTION			Carbohydrate g	9.3	Of which saturates g	0.9	Salt g	0.7
Energy kcal		106	Of which sugars g	8.2	Fibre g	1.9	Portion fruit and veg	2

Lasagne

Serves: 4 or 6   **Prep:** 15 minutes (not Ragu)   **Cook:** 45 minutes
500kcal and 14.4g Fat per ¼ recipe; 320kcal and 9.6g Fat per ⅙ recipe

Lasagne needn't be off-limits on a diet if you make it with lower-fat ingredients.
This one uses the Ragu recipe (page 166) and a white sauce made without added
fat.

1 quantity of Ragu –
   see page 166
600ml 1% Fat milk
2 bay leaves
50g cornflour
Black pepper
Grated nutmeg
120g dry lasagne
50g grated
   parmesan

1. **Make the Ragu.**
2. **Preheat oven to 190°C/170°C Fan/GM5.**
3. **Place 500ml of the milk and the bay leaves in a non-stick pan, bring gradually to simmering point, and allow to simmer slowly for 5 or so minutes.**
4. **Mix the remaining milk with the cornflour and stir into the hot milk, and allow to thicken, stirring all the time. Remove from the heat, take out the bay leaves and stir in some black pepper and some grated nutmeg. This is your white sauce.**

Serves 4

NUTRITIONAL ANALYSIS PER PORTION		Protein g	40.5	Fat g	14.4	Sodium g	0.3
		Carbohydrate g	50.5	Of which saturates g	6.5	Salt g	0.75
Energy kcal	500	Of which sugars g	14.3	Fibre g	3.7	Portion fruit and veg	1

Serves 6

NUTRITIONAL ANALYSIS PER PORTION		Protein g	24.2	Fat g	9.6	Sodium g	0.2
		Carbohydrate g	30.8	Of which saturates g	4.3	Salt g	0.5
Energy kcal	320	Of which sugars g	9	Fibre g	2.7	Portion fruit and veg	1

5. Spread half of the ragu on the base of a lasagne dish and spoon over about one-third of the white sauce.
6. Cover with a few pasta sheets and then spoon over the remaining ragu. Cover with the last pasta sheets.
7. Pour over the remaining white sauce and sprinkle over the parmesan.
8. Bake for 40–45 minutes until the pasta is cooked through and the lasagne is golden brown.
9. Serve hot.

Serving Suggestions: Serve with a large green salad and crusty bread.

Storage: Can be kept in the fridge, covered with cling film, for 2–3 days. Can also be frozen.

Pasta Sauce
with Mediterranean Vegetables

Serves: 4   **Prep:** 5 minutes   **Cook:** 30 minutes

88kcal and 4.8g fat per serving

This is an easy sauce, which is ready and on the table in half an hour. It is suitable for all the family – even those who turn up their noses at courgettes, as these are disguised by blitzing the sauce with a hand blender. You may like to leave out the black olives until you have blended the sauce, then pop them in for the last few minutes to heat through.

1 tbsp olive oil

1 medium onion, finely chopped

1 clove garlic, crushed

150g (1 large) courgette

600g tomatoes, roughly chopped

25g tomato purée

1 tsp sugar

150ml water

50g pitted black olives

Black pepper

1 dsp chopped fresh or 1 tsp dried oregano

1. In a non-stick saucepan heat the oil and gently fry the onion and garlic.
2. Grate the courgette and add to the pan, continue to heat for 5–10 minutes until softened.
3. Add the tomatoes, tomato purée and sugar.
4. Pour in the water and olives. If preferred leave olives out until after the sauce is cooked and blended.
5. Bring to the boil, cover and simmer for 20 minutes. Add the black pepper and the oregano.
6. Lightly blend to make a sauce with a few chunks. Add the olives if not already included.
7. Serve with pasta and a salad of leaves.

Serving Suggestions: Served with 75g rigatoni and 10g grated parmesan: 400kcal and 9.3g fat.

Storage: The sauce can be stored in the fridge for 2–3 days. It can also be frozen.

NUTRITIONAL ANALYSIS PER PORTION		Protein g	2.7	Fat g	4.8	Sodium g	300
		Carbohydrate g	9.4	Of which saturates g	0.8	Salt g	0.75
Kcal	88	Of which sugars g	8.3	Fibre g	2.0	Portion fruit and veg	2

Salmon and Asparagus Linguine

Serves: 2   **Prep:** 5 minutes   **Cook:** 15 minutes

500kcal and 13.3g fat per portion

Salmon is a source of essential fatty acids, which have numerous health bene-fits. Oily fish, like salmon, is recommended to be eaten at least once a week as part of a healthy diet, so this is an ideal way of enjoying it.

150g wholewheat linguine or spaghetti

150g salmon fillet

50ml white wine

1 tbsp fresh lemon juice

1 bay leaf

200g asparagus

150g Quark

1 tsp chopped fresh dill

1. Cook the pasta according to the packet instructions.
2. Meanwhile place the salmon in a small non-stick saucepan and add the wine, lemon juice and bay leaf. Poach the salmon by heating gently until the fish flakes.
3. Steam the asparagus while the salmon is cooking.
4. Remove the salmon from the heat and stir in the Quark and dill. This will also break up the salmon.
5. Stir in the asparagus and pasta, and serve at once.

Serving Suggestions: Serve with a crisp leaf salad.

Storage: Not suitable for storage.

NUTRITIONAL ANALYSIS		Protein g	38.2	Fat g	13.3	Sodium g	0.2
PER PORTION		Carbohydrate g	54.8	Of which saturates g	3.2	Salt g	0.5
Energy kcal	500	Of which sugars g	7.6	Fibre g	7.7	Portion fruit and veg	1

Spaghetti with Chilli Prawns

Serves: 2   **Prep:** 5 minutes   **Cook:** 10 minutes

450kcal and 13g fat per portion

This recipe is so quick and easy it will become a weekday favourite. You can add other vegetables such as baby corn or petits pois instead of the mangetout, and if you don't like chilli, simply leave it out.

150g spaghetti

160g mangetout, trimmed

2 tbsp olive oil

1 bird's eye chilli, finely chopped

250g cooked peeled king prawns

Grated zest of 1 lemon

20ml lemon juice (½ a lemon)

1. Boil the pasta according to the packet instructions. In the last couple of minutes add the mangetout and cook until they are just beginning to become tender (2–3 minutes).

2. When the pasta is nearly cooked, place the oil in a wok or non-stick pan and fry the chilli and prawns.

3. As soon as the prawns are piping hot, remove from the heat and stir in the lemon juice and zest.

4. Drain the pasta and mangetout, and place it in a serving bowl.

5. Pour over the prawns and cooking juices.

6. Serve at once.

Serving Suggestions: Serve with a glass of chilled white wine and a crisp salad.

Storage: If you like pasta salad, chill and use for a packed lunch. Not suitable for freezing.

NUTRITIONAL ANALYSIS PER PORTION		Protein g	32.3	Fat g	13	Sodium g	0.6
		Carbohydrate g	54	Of which saturates g	2.2	Salt g	1.5
Energy kcal	450	Of which sugars g	5	Fibre g	3.6	Portion fruit and veg	1

Spinach and Mushroom Pasta Bake

Serves: 2 Prep: 10 minutes Cook: 20 minutes

410kcal and 11.7g fat per portion

This is a great way to eat vegetables – all wrapped up in a delicious sauce with pasta.

1 tbsp olive oil

40g (2) shallots, finely chopped

100g mushrooms, sliced

200g chopped canned tomatoes

5 basil leaves, torn

150g pasta, such as rigatoni or penne

70g young spinach leaves, washed and drained

Black pepper

30g parmesan cheese, grated

1. Preheat oven to 200°C/180°C Fan/GM6.
2. Heat the oil in a large non-stick saucepan and gently fry the shallots until softened.
3. Stir in the mushrooms, tomatoes and basil leaves, and bring to the boil. Reduce the heat and simmer for 10 minutes.
4. Meanwhile cook the pasta according to the packet instructions and drain.
5. When the pasta is cooked, stir the spinach leaves into the sauce and then mix with the drained pasta. Grind over black pepper to taste.
6. Spoon the mixture into an ovenproof dish and sprinkle over the parmesan cheese.
7. Place in the oven for 10 minutes until the cheese is browned. Serve at once.

Serving Suggestions: Why not serve with a glass of orange juice – or even red wine?

Storage: Best served at once, but you could refrigerate for 24 hours before baking.

NUTRITIONAL ANALYSIS		Protein g	17.4	Fat g	11.7	Sodium g	0.3
PER PORTION		Carbohydrate g	59.3	Of which saturates g	4.3	Salt g	0.75
Energy kcal	410	Of which sugars g	6.7	Fibre g	4.8	Portion fruit and veg	2

Butternut Squash and Bacon with Wholemeal Spaghetti

Serves: 4 **Prep:** 4 minutes **Cook:** 15 minutes

445kcal and 15g fat per portion

Although streaky bacon is quite fatty, the small amount used here really adds to this recipe. If you can't get hold of fresh butternut squash, look for frozen squash in the supermarket (Waitrose stocks it).

1 butternut squash (about 800g)

300g wholemeal spaghetti

120g streaky bacon, cubed

3 cloves garlic, crushed

2 tbsp olive oil

1 heaped tsp chopped fresh thyme

Black pepper

1. Halve the squash lengthwise and scoop out the seeds.
2. Either cover with cling film and cook in the microwave for about 7–8 minutes on 800W, or bake in the oven for 45 minutes at 200°C/180°C Fan/GM6 until the flesh is tender.
3. Cook the pasta for 10–12 minutes, then drain.
4. Place the bacon in a non-stick pan and heat gently to release the fat and make it crispy.
5. Stir in the garlic.
6. When the squash is softened, scoop out the flesh with a spoon and add it to the pan with the bacon, stirring often. The flesh will break down a bit in the pan, but leave some as chunks.
7. Add the oil, thyme and black pepper.
8. Serve the spaghetti with the sauce while it is piping hot.

Serving Suggestions: Serve with a green salad or steamed sugar snaps.

Storage: Not suitable for storage.

NUTRITIONAL ANALYSIS PER PORTION		Protein g	17.3	Fat g	15	Sodium g	0.5
		Carbohydrate g	64.5	Of which saturates g	3.8	Salt g	–
Energy kcal	445	Of which sugars g	6.9	Fibre g	3.8	Portion fruit and veg	1

Sauces, Dressings and Dips

Apple and Mint Dressing

Serves: 4   **Prep:** 5 minutes

27kcal and 0g fat per portion

A fat-free dressing that tastes delicious with leaves, especially watercress or spinach. You can also try it as a marinade for pork.

50ml unsweetened cloudy apple juice

15ml (1 tbsp) cider or white wine vinegar

16g (2 level tsp) runny honey

1 tbsp chopped fresh mint

1. **Place all the ingredients in a jar and shake together.**
2. **Chill until required.**

Serving Suggestions: Serve with spinach, rocket and watercress salad leaves.

Storage: Store for 2–3 days in the fridge.

NUTRITIONAL ANALYSIS		Protein g	0.1	Fat g	0	Sodium g	0
PER PORTION		Carbohydrate g	6.6	Of which saturates g	0	Salt g	0
Energy kcal	27	Of which sugars g	6.5	Fibre g	0	Portion fruit and veg	0

Tomato and Coriander Salsa

Serves: 4   **Prep:** 5 minutes

13kcal and 0.2g fat per portion

Whiz up these fresh ingredients in a blender or food processor for a quick and easy low-fat dip, or as a sauce to accompany burgers, grilled meat or fish.

260g ripe tomatoes

1 clove garlic, peeled

20g fresh coriander

1 tbsp fresh lemon or lime juice

Black pepper

1. **Wash the tomatoes and cut into quarters.**
2. **Place all the ingredients in a food processor and blend to make a slightly chunky salsa.**
3. **Serve at once, or cover with cling film and chill until required.**

Serving Suggestions: Serve with carrot or celery sticks for a low-fat snack, or with Pork Patties (page 161).

Storage: Can be stored for a day in the fridge but will lose its vitamin-C content if not eaten quickly.

NUTRITIONAL ANALYSIS		Protein g	0.7	Fat g	0.2	Sodium mg	Trace
PER PORTION		Carbohydrate g	2.1	Of which saturates g	0.1	Salt g	Trace
Energy kcal	13	Of which sugars g	2	Fibre g	0.7	Portion fruit and veg	1

Blueberry and Orange Coulis

Serves: 4　　**Prep:** 5 minutes　　**Cook:** 15 minutes
50kcal and 0.1g Fat per portion

A simple sauce to liven up ice cream, pancakes or simply serve with yogurt.

200g blueberries

Zest and juice of
　1 medium orange

25g sugar (optional)

1. **Place the blueberries in a small pan and gently heat, stirring occasionally, for about 10 minutes until they have popped and are softened.**
2. **Stir in the grated orange zest and juice, and heat through for another minute.**
3. **Taste the coulis and if it is not sweet enough add the sugar, and heat gently to dissolve. Do not allow to boil.**
4. **Remove from the heat and allow to cool to room temperature.**

Serving Suggestions: Serve for breakfast with Buttermilk Pancakes (page 68), or with a pot of fat-free plain yogurt.

Storage: May be stored in an airtight container for 2–3 days. Can also be frozen.

NUTRITIONAL ANALYSIS		Protein g	0.6	Fat g	0.1	Sodium g	Trace
PER PORTION		Carbohydrate g	11.9	Of which saturates g	0	Salt g	Trace
Energy kcal	50	Of which sugars g	11.9	Fibre g	1.4	Portion fruit and veg	1

Chilli and Coriander Dressing

Serves: 4   **Prep:** 2 minutes

29kcal and 0.1g fat per portion

A simple salad dressing that is guaranteed to liven up any salad. There are lots of sweet chilli dipping sauces available in the supermarket. The nutrition information on this one was based on Blue Dragon sweet chilli dipping sauce with kaffir lime leaves.

50ml sweet chilli dipping sauce

50ml fresh lime or lemon juice

1 tbsp freshly chopped coriander leaves

1. **Place all the ingredients in a jam jar and shake to mix.**
2. **Chill until required.**

Serving Suggestions: Add crushed fresh garlic or ginger root to give this a real zing.

Storage: Can be stored for 2 days maximum in the fridge.

NUTRITIONAL ANALYSIS		Protein g	0.2	Fat g	0.1	Sodium g	0.2
PER PORTION		Carbohydrate g	7	Of which saturates g	0	Salt g	0.5
Energy kcal	29	Of which sugars g	6.9	Fibre g	0.3	Portion fruit and veg	0

Chive Dip

Serves: 6   **Prep:** 5 minutes

36kcal and 2.1g fat per portion

This is a very basic dip that you can adapt by adding other herbs. You can also try it as a simple sauce when serving fish such as salmon. Some carrot sticks and chive dip will take the edge off your appetite while you are preparing supper, or in between meals.

140g carton half-fat sour cream

150g virtually fat-free fromage frais

1 tbsp snipped chives

Black pepper

Grated zest of ½ a lemon (optional)

1. Mix all the ingredients together in a bowl.
2. Cover and chill until required.

Serving Suggestions: Served with 1 small carrot (60g) and 1 small stick of celery (30g): 60kcal and 2.4g fat. Served with 2 average breadsticks (7g each): 95kcal and 3.2g fat.

Storage: Can be stored in the fridge for 3 days in an airtight container.

NUTRITIONAL ANALYSIS		Protein g	1.9	Fat g	2.1	Sodium g	Trace
PER PORTION		Carbohydrate g	2.3	Of which saturates g	1.3	Salt g	Trace
Energy kcal	36	Of which sugars g	1.7	Fibre g	Trace	Portion fruit and veg	0

Fat-free Yogurt and Herb Dressing

Serves: 8 tbsp   **Prep:** 5 minutes

16kcal and <0.1g fat per portion

You can use your favourite herb in this recipe, or whatever is in season.

200g fat-free plain yogurt

Grated zest of 1 lime

5g (1 tsp) sugar

1 dsp fresh lemon or lime juice

1 tbsp fresh mixed herbs, e.g. tarragon, parsley, chervil

1. **Mix all the ingredients in a bottle and chill.**

Serving Suggestions: Try with a leaf salad, or watercress mixed with cucumber.

Storage: Will keep in the fridge for 2–3 days. Not suitable for freezing.

NUTRITIONAL ANALYSIS		Protein g	1.3	Fat g	0.1	Sodium g	0
PER PORTION		Carbohydrate g	2.6	Of which saturates g	0	Salt g	0
Energy kcal	16	Of which sugars g	2.5	Fibre g	0	Portion fruit and veg	0

Home-made Houmous

Serves: 4   **Prep:** 5 minutes

123kcal and 7.3g fat per portion

Making your own houmous is so easy you will wonder why you never did it before. Instead of the high-fat version sold in the shops, you can use minimal oil and lots of lemon juice to make a delicious lower-fat version.

400g can chickpeas in water, drained and rinsed

20g (1 level tbsp) tahini paste

Juice of 1 lemon

1 clove garlic

1 tbsp olive oil

Black pepper

1. Place all the ingredients in a blender and whiz until smooth.
2. Add a little water if the mixture is a bit stiff.
3. Chill and serve.

Serving Suggestions: Serve with carrot, celery or pepper sticks. You can alter the ingredients and leave the nutrition the same by swapping the olive oil for 1 tbsp (30g) of sundried tomato paste.

Storage: Store for up to 3 days in the fridge in an airtight container.

NUTRITIONAL ANALYSIS PER PORTION		Protein g	5.3	Fat g	7.3	Sodium mg	Trace
		Carbohydrate g	9	Of which saturates g	1	Salt g	Trace
Energy kcal	123	Of which sugars g	0.4	Fibre g	0.5	Portion fruit and veg	½

Pineapple Salsa

Serves: 2   **Prep:** 5 minutes
46kcal and 0.2g fat per portion

Rich in vitamin C, this salsa livens up chicken, pork or turkey. A can of pineapple in juice can be substituted if you can't buy fresh.

160g (2 slices) fresh pineapple, roughly cubed

25g (3 medium) mild peppadew peppers

2g (1 sprig) lemon thyme

1. **Place the pineapple in a food processor along with the peppers and thyme.**
2. **Blitz for a few seconds to make a chunky salsa.**
3. **Chill or serve at once.**

Serving Suggestions: Try with Turkey Steaks with Crumb and Sundried Tomato Topping (page 119).

Storage: Can be stored for up to 2 days in the fridge in an airtight container.

NUTRITIONAL ANALYSIS		Protein g	0.4	Fat g	0.2	Sodium g	Trace
PER PORTION		Carbohydrate g	10.6	Of which saturates g	0	Salt g	Trace
Energy kcal	46	Of which sugars g	10.5	Fibre g	2	Portion fruit and veg	1

Pomegranate Sauce

Serves: 4   **Prep:** 5 minutes   **Cook:** 20 minutes
60kcal and 1g fat per portion

This sauce looks beautiful – its deep red colour underlies its excellent nutritional state. Pomegranate, like red wine, is full of protective antioxidants, but some can be damaged by overheating, so don't boil the pomegranate, just heat gently.

1 small red onion,
  finely chopped
1 tsp olive oil
200ml chicken stock
100ml red wine
10ml (1 dsp) balsamic
  vinegar
10g (1 dsp) sugar
1 tsp chopped lemon
  thyme
150g pomegranate
  seeds

1. Fry the onion in the olive oil until softened, about 5 minutes.
2. Stir in the stock, wine, vinegar, sugar and thyme, and bring to the boil.
3. Boil for 10 minutes to reduce the volume by about half.
4. Add the pomegranate seeds and warm through.
5. Serve at once.

Serving Suggestions: Try with grilled steak, ostrich or venison.

Storage: Can be refrigerated for 2 days.

NUTRITIONAL ANALYSIS		Protein g	0.7	Fat g	1	Sodium g	0.1
PER PORTION		Carbohydrate g	8.5	Of which saturates g	0.2	Salt g	0.25
Energy kcal	60	Of which sugars g	8.5	Fibre g	1.5	Portion fruit and veg	½

Raita

Serves: 4   **Prep:** 5 minutes
23kcal and 0.1g fat per portion

A superb foil to hot curries or dhals, raita is simple to make and this version almost fat-free.

1 tbsp chopped fresh mint

150g fat-free Greek yogurt

150g cucumber

Black pepper

½ tsp toasted cumin seeds (optional)

1. Mix the mint and yogurt together.
2. Coarsely grate the cucumber and place in a sieve. Press out as much liquid as you can before mixing into the yogurt/mint mixture.
3. Season with black pepper and, if you like, the cumin seeds.
4. Chill until ready to serve.

Serving Suggestions: Serve with Asian dishes or as a dip with pitta bread.

Storage: Will keep in an airtight container in the fridge for up to 2 days. Cannot be frozen.

NUTRITIONAL ANALYSIS		Protein g	3.6	Fat g	0.1	Sodium g	Trace
PER PORTION		Carbohydrate g	2	Of which saturates g	0	Salt g	Trace
Energy kcal	23	Of which sugars g	1.9	Fibre g	0.2	Portion fruit and veg	½

Raspberry Salsa

Serves: 2   **Prep:** 2 minutes
33kcal and 0.3g fat per portion

For summer days when you are grilling chicken or pork, this simple salsa adds a fruity touch. You can use frozen raspberries if you like.

150g fresh raspberries

1 tsp demerara sugar

1 tsp balsamic vinegar, white if possible

2 tsp chopped lemon thyme

1. **Place the raspberries in a bowl and crush lightly with a fork.**
2. **Add the sugar, vinegar and thyme, and mix.**
3. **Chill until serving.**

Serving Suggestions: Serve with grilled pork or chicken or to accompany a plain leaf salad.

Storage: Keep in the fridge for 24 hours only. Not suitable for freezing.

NUTRITIONAL ANALYSIS		Protein g	1.1	Fat g	0.3	Sodium g	Trace
PER PORTION		Carbohydrate g	6.9	Of which saturates g	0.1	Salt g	Trace
Energy kcal	33	Of which sugars g	6.7	Fibre g	1.9	Portion fruit and veg	1

Smoked Trout Paté

Serves: 3   **Prep:** 5 minutes
125kcal and 4.9g fat per portion

This paté can also be served as a dip. Smoked salmon could also be used instead of the trout.

120g smoked trout

200g extra-light soft cheese

Grated zest and juice of ½ a lime

Black pepper

1. **Place the trout, soft cheese and lime zest in a small food-processor bowl. Pulse to make a soft mixture with a few lumps.**

2. **Add the lime juice and black pepper, and pulse again just to mix.**

3. **Place in serving dishes and chill until required.**

Serving Suggestions: Serve with oatcakes or with salad leaves and a lightly blanched slice of fennel.

Storage: Will keep refrigerated for 3 days, but unsuitable for freezing.

NUTRITIONAL ANALYSIS		Protein g	17.9	Fat g	4.9	Sodium g	0.5
PER PORTION		Carbohydrate g	2.8	Of which saturates g	2.3	Salt g	1.25
Energy kcal	125	Of which sugars g	2.4	Fibre g	Trace	Portion fruit and veg	0

Spicy Harissa Dressing

Serves: 4   **Prep:** 5 minutes

30kcal and 2.8g fat per portion

Harissa is a paste made from a range of different ingredients but based on spices, chillies and tomatoes in oil. A little goes a long way, so although it is high in fat you will only need a very small amount. An alternative harissa, if you can't find it, would be your favourite curry paste.

1 level tbsp harissa
dressing

150g pot fat-free
Greek yogurt

1. **Mix the harissa and yogurt, and serve, chilled.**

Serving Suggestions: Use as a dip with carrot sticks.

Storage: Can be stored, covered in the fridge, for 2 days. Not suitable for freezing.

NUTRITIONAL ANALYSIS PER PORTION		Protein g	3.3	Fat g	2.8	Sodium g	Unknown
		Carbohydrate g	1.4	Of which saturates g	0.3	Salt g	Unknown
Energy kcal	30	Of which sugars g	1.4	Fibre g	Trace	Portion fruit and veg	0

Sweetcorn Salsa

Serves: 4   **Prep:** 5 minutes   **Cook:** 5 minutes
30kcal and 0.3g fat per portion

Sweet and spicy, this salsa is great for summer barbecues, or to give plain grilled chicken a zing.

220g sweetcorn, canned or frozen, thawed

1 tsp grated fresh ginger

50g peppadew peppers

60g spring onions, sliced

1 tbsp fresh coriander leaves, chopped

Black pepper

1. **Cook the sweetcorn (if frozen) for 2–3 minutes. Drain the sweetcorn in a sieve and press to remove as much liquid as you can.**
2. **Place the sweetcorn, ginger, peppers and spring onions in a food processor and lightly blitz so that the ingredients are just chopped.**
3. **Remove from the processor and stir in the coriander and black pepper to taste.**
4. **Chill until required.**

Serving Suggestions: Serve as a dip with toasted pitta bread or with barbecued meat.

Storage: Will keep in the fridge for 2 days in an airtight container. Not suitable for freezing.

NUTRITIONAL ANALYSIS		Protein g	1.7	Fat g	0.3	Sodium g	Trace
PER PORTION		Carbohydrate g	5.2	Of which saturates g	0	Salt g	Trace
Energy kcal	30	Of which sugars g	4.7	Fibre g	1.2	Portion fruit and veg	2

Bitter Chocolate Sauce

Serves: 6   **Prep:** 5 minutes   **Cook:** 10 minutes

70kcal and 2.4g fat per portion (with cream);
50kcal and 0.9g fat (without cream)

If you like dark chocolate, then this is for you. This delicious sauce uses best-quality cocoa for a glossy but low-fat sauce. If you want very low fat, miss out the cream.

50g dark brown or
   muscovado sugar
25g good-quality
   cocoa powder
150ml water
15g (1 level tbsp)
   arrowroot
100ml reduced-fat
   sour cream

1. **Place the sugar and cocoa powder in a small saucepan, and gradually whisk in the water, making sure it mixes properly.**
2. **Bring to simmering point, then remove from the heat.**
3. **Mix the arrowroot with another 50ml of water and stir into the sauce. Heat until the sauce is slightly thickened.**
4. **Now stir in the sour cream and heat for another couple of minutes.**
5. **Cool and store until needed.**

Serving Suggestions: Serve with poached fruit, such as pears, or baked bananas.

Storage: Will keep for up to 1 week in an airtight container in the fridge.

With cream

NUTRITIONAL ANALYSIS PER PORTION		Protein g	1.5	Fat g	2.4	Sodium g	Trace
		Carbohydrate g	11.4	Of which saturates g	1.4	Salt g	Trace
Energy kcal	70	Of which sugars g	8.9	Fibre g	0	Portion fruit and veg	0

Without cream

NUTRITIONAL ANALYSIS PER PORTION		Protein g	0.8	Fat g	0.9	Sodium g	Trace
		Carbohydrate g	10.4	Of which saturates g	0.5	Salt g	Trace
Energy kcal	50	Of which sugars g	8.4	Fibre g	0	Portion fruit and veg	0

Desserts

Apple and Cranberry Crisp

Serves: 6   **Prep:** 10 minutes   **Cook:** 35–40 minutes
238kcal and 7.9g Fat per serving

This homely dessert has a crumble-type topping that uses crunchy oat cereal as well as oats. If you can't get dried cranberries you can always substitute the same amount of raisins or chopped dried apricots.

640g (2 large) cooking apples

50g dried sweetened cranberries

50g sugar

120g rolled (porridge) oats

50g demerara sugar

50g soft butter or sunflower spread

80g crunchy oat cereal

1. Preheat oven to 190°C/170°C Fan/GM5.
2. Peel and core the apples, cut into slices and place in an ovenproof dish.
3. Sprinkle over the cranberries and sugar.
4. To make the topping, mix together the oats and demerara sugar and, using a fork, mix in the butter.
5. Stir in the crunchy oat cereal and spoon over the fruit.
6. Bake for 35–40 minutes until the topping is golden brown.

Serving Suggestions: Served with 1 tbsp of low-fat yogurt: 265kcal and 8.6g fat.

Storage: Best served straight away, but will keep in the fridge for 2 days. Can be frozen.

NUTRITIONAL ANALYSIS PER PORTION		Protein g	3.7	Fat g	7.9	Sodium mg	51
		Carbohydrate g	50.9	Of which saturates g	1.9	Salt g	0.1
Kcal	238	Of which sugars g	31.9	Fibre g	2.6	Portion fruit and veg	1

Summer Fruit Compote

Serves: 2 **Prep:** 5 minutes **Cook:** 5 minutes
125kcal and 0.5g fat per portion

Rich in vitamin C, this delicious compote makes a simple dessert, which you can also use as a sauce with pancakes or to sweeten yogurt.

250g frozen summer fruits, thawed

100ml hedgerow cordial or similar fruit cordial

1 heaped tsp arrowroot

1. **Place the fruits and any thawed juice in a saucepan and gently heat.**
2. **Stir the cordial into the arrowroot and pour into the pan.**
3. **Allow to come just to boiling point and simmer for 1–2 minutes until the sauce has thickened.**
4. **Remove from the heat and cool.**

Serving Suggestions: A delicious dessert alone, or try for breakfast with Buttermilk Pancakes (page 68). 1 tbsp (40g) provides 38kcal and 0.2g fat.

Storage: Refrigerate for 2–3 days. Can be frozen – stir well when thawed.

NUTRITIONAL ANALYSIS PER PORTION		Protein g	1.7	Fat g	0.5	Sodium g	Trace
		Carbohydrate g	30.4	Of which saturates g	0	Salt g	Trace
Energy kcal	125	Of which sugars g	8.9	Fibre g	4.1	Portion fruit and veg	2

Autumn Fruit Salad

Serves: 4   **Prep:** 10 minutes
100kcal and 0.3g fat per portion

In October and November, as you enjoy watching the leaves turn, make the most of the seasonal fruits around you. Like the autumn leaves, this salad is rich orange and red in colour, and is also full of protective plant substances and vitamins.

150g pomegranate seeds or
1 pomegranate, seeded
200g red grapes, washed
1 large ripe pear – (about 200–250g)
110g (2) ripe figs, washed, trimmed and cut into segments
1 Sharon fruit, fully ripe

1. Place the pomegranate seeds in a large serving bowl and add the grapes, halving them if they are particularly large.
2. Peel the pear, remove the core and dice into small pieces, and add to the bowl.
3. Stir in the figs.
4. Remove the top of the Sharon fruit and scoop out the ripe flesh with a spoon. Mash or chop the flesh slightly to break it up, then stir into the fruit salad.
5. Serve at once. If you need to make this in advance, make sure that it reaches room temperature before serving.

Serving Suggestions: A few tbsp of ginger wine or cordial will add a zing.

Storage: Store in the fridge in an airtight container for 2 days.

NUTRITIONAL ANALYSIS		Protein g	1.4	Fat g	0.3	Sodium g	Trace
PER PORTION		Carbohydrate g	22.7	Of which saturates g	Trace	Salt g	Trace
Energy kcal	100	Of which sugars g	22.7	Fibre g	3.6	Portion fruit and veg	2

Baked Peaches with Amaretti Filling

Serves: 2 **Prep:** 5 minutes **Cook:** 20–30 minutes

155kcal and 1.3g fat per portion

In the summer these baked peaches will remind you of holidays spent in Italy. Ratafia biscuits can be used instead of amaretti biscuits.

32g (about 6) amaretti biscuits, crushed lightly

10g (2 level tsp) runny honey

2 tbsp marsala or sweet white wine

2 large ripe but firm peaches, halved and stones removed

1. Preheat oven to 190°C/170°C Fan/GM5.
2. Mix the crushed biscuits with the honey and 1 tablespoon of the wine.
3. Pile the mixture into the hollow in the peach left by the stone, and place in an ovenproof dish.
4. Sprinkle over a little more wine and bake for 20–30 minutes until the peaches are soft.
5. Serve at room temperature.

Serving Suggestions: Served with 1 level tbsp half-fat crème fraîche: 182kcal and 4.1g fat.

Storage: May be kept for 24 hours in the fridge. Bring to room temperature before serving.

NUTRITIONAL ANALYSIS PER PORTION		Protein g	2.4	Fat g	1.3	Sodium g	Trace
		Carbohydrate g	30.7	Of which saturates g	0.1	Salt g	Trace
Energy kcal	155	Of which sugars g	29.4	Fibre g	2.3	Portion fruit and veg	1

Baked Plums with Port

Serves: 2   **Prep:** 5–10 minutes   **Cook:** 30 minutes

158kcal and 0.2g fat per portion

This is so easy and so tasty. It even freezes, so if you happen to have a plum tree or are given a lot of plums in the early autumn you can make extra and keep it for the depths of winter.

300g plums of your choice

120g (1 small) orange

25g demerara sugar

½ tsp ground cinnamon

50ml port

1. **Preheat oven to 180°C/160°C Fan/GM4.**
2. **Halve the plums, remove the stones and place the plums in an ovenproof dish.**
3. **Using a potato peeler, cut a few strips of zest from the orange and add to the plums. Then squeeze the orange juice over the plums.**
4. **Sprinkle over the sugar and cinnamon, and, lastly, pour over the port.**
5. **Place in the oven and bake for 30 minutes or until the fruit is soft but not collapsed.**
6. **Remove the orange zest and serve warm or at room temperature.**

Serving Suggestions: Served with Vanilla 'Cream' (page 271): 225kcal and 1.6g fat. If you don't want to use port, just use 50ml more fresh orange juice.

Storage: Can be kept in the fridge for a day or two, or may be frozen.

NUTRITIONAL ANALYSIS PER PORTION		Protein g	1.2	Fat g	0.2	Sodium g	Trace
		Carbohydrate g	30.9	Of which saturates g	Trace	Salt g	Trace
Energy kcal	158	Of which sugars g	30.9	Fibre g	2.7	Portion fruit and veg	1

Bramley and Mango Brûlée

Serves: 4   **Prep:** 15 minutes   **Cook:** 15 minutes
120kcal and 0.2g fat per portion

A base of delicious apple and mango with a very low-fat topping and a crunchy crust. One small brûlée provides just over 100kcal, so you can treat yourself to this dessert once in a while.

300 Bramley apples, peeled, cored and diced

2 tsp sugar (optional)

150g (1 medium) ripe mango, cubed

20ml lemon juice (juice of ½ a lemon)

200g pot virtually fat-free fromage frais

40g demerara sugar

1. Place the apples in a saucepan with 2 tablespoons of water. Cover and cook over a low heat until the apples are mushy. Taste and, if sour, add the sugar. Allow to cool.

2. Blitz the mango cubes in a food processor and mix with the cooled apple and the lemon juice.

3. Spoon into 4 ramekin dishes.

4. Stir the fromage frais and spoon over the fruit. Smooth the top.

5. Sprinkle over the demerara sugar.

6. Use a culinary blowtorch to caramelize the sugar, or place under a preheated hot grill until the sugar is bubbling and golden brown.

7. Serve either at once or chill until required.

Serving Suggestions: Instead of mango, use all apple, or replace with blackberries or blueberries.

Storage: Will keep in the fridge for 24 hours. Not suitable for freezing.

NUTRITIONAL ANALYSIS	Protein g	4.4	Fat g	0.2	Sodium g	Trace
PER PORTION	Carbohydrate g	27.9	Of which saturates g	0.1	Salt g	Trace
Energy kcal	120	Of which sugars g	27.7	Fibre g	2.7	Portion fruit and veg	1

Fruits of the Forest Mousse

Serves: 4   **Prep:** 10 minutes

50kcal and 0.1g fat per portion

This recipe is a sister one to the Fruits of the Forest Soufflé (page 261) and is designed so you can make both at once, saving this one for later. The recipe here is the full recipe, but if you are using half the soufflé mixture, just halve the amount of gelatine.

250g fruits of the forest, such as blackberries, blackcurrants, raspberries

25g caster sugar

2 level tsp gelatine

50ml hot water

2 egg whites

1. **Heat the fruit with the sugar for 2–3 minutes just to dissolve the sugar, stirring occasionally. Cool and blend.**

2. **Push the mixture through a sieve with a spoon, saving the purée and discarding the seeds.**

3. **Dissolve the gelatine in the hot water and pour into the fruit purée. Allow to cool for a few minutes.**

4. **Whisk the egg whites and fold in the fruit purée.**

5. **Pour into a serving dish and chill.**

Serving Suggestions: Served with 1 rounded tbsp (40g) fat-free Greek yogurt: 70kcal and 0.1g fat.

Storage: Refrigerate for up to 3 days. Not suitable for freezing.

NUTRITIONAL ANALYSIS PER PORTION	Protein g	3.1	Fat g	0.1	Sodium mg	Trace
	Carbohydrate g	10	Of which saturates g	0	Salt g	Trace
Energy kcal 50	Of which sugars g	10	Fibre g	1	Portion fruit and veg	½

Fruits of the Forest Soufflé

Serves: 4   **Prep:** 10 minutes   **Cook:** 12 minutes

50kcal and 0.1g fat per portion

This is the world's easiest soufflé, which will rise to your expectations both physically and in taste. The mixture is sufficiently versatile to become the basis of the Fruits of the Forest Mousse (page 260), so if you don't need 4 portions, make the other pudding at the same time for the next day.

250g fruits of the forest, such as blackberries, blackcurrants, raspberries

25g caster sugar

2 egg whites

Icing sugar

1. **Preheat oven to 200°C/180°C Fan/GM6.**
2. **Heat the fruit with the sugar for 2–3 minutes to just dissolve the sugar, stirring occasionally. Cool and blend.**
3. **Push the mixture through a sieve with a spoon, saving the purée and discarding the seeds.**
4. **Whisk the egg whites and fold in the fruit purée.**
5. **Pour into 4 ramekins and bake for 12 minutes until risen and set.**
6. **Sprinkle lightly with icing sugar, and serve at once.**

Serving Suggestions: Eat at once!

Storage: While soufflés do not normally keep, you may find you can reheat this one in a microwave on High for 15–20 seconds and watch it rise. Only keep in the fridge for 1 day.

NUTRITIONAL ANALYSIS	Protein g	2.1	Fat g	0.1	Sodium g	Trace
PER PORTION		Carbohydrate g	10.3	Of which saturates g	0	Salt g	Trace
Energy kcal	50	Of which sugars g	10.3	Fibre g	2	Portion fruit and veg	½

Mango and Kiwi Salad
with Blackcurrant Sorbet

Serves: 1   **Prep:** 5 minutes

117kcal and 0.4g fat per portion

This simple fruit salad is very colourful and full of vitamin C from the kiwi fruit and blackcurrant, as well as essential vitamin A from the mango.

1 kiwi fruit

100g mango cubes

1 scoop (65g)
blackcurrant
sorbet

1. **Peel and slice the kiwi fruit.**

2. **Mix the mango and kiwi together.**

3. **Serve with the sorbet.**

Serving Suggestions: Substitute the blackcurrant sorbet for lemon or mango, checking nutrition information.

Storage: Best eaten straight away!

NUTRITIONAL ANALYSIS						
PER PORTION	Protein g	1.3	Fat g	0.4	Sodium mg	Trace
	Carbohydrate g	28	Of which saturates g	0.1	Salt g	Trace
Energy kcal	117	Of which sugars g	27.6	Fibre g	4	Portion fruit and veg	2

Mango Fool

Serves: 4   **Prep:** 5 minutes
110kcal and 0.6g fat per portion

A simply delicious smooth dessert high in essential vitamin A, which uses ready-made custard to save you time. Also look out for cans of pure mango purée in the supermarket.

210g (half-can) low-fat ready-made custard

320g mango purée

150g tub fat-free Greek yogurt

Finely grated zest of 1 lime

1. **Mix the custard and the mango purée in a bowl.**
2. **Stir in the yogurt and lime zest.**
3. **Pour into individual serving dishes.**
4. **Chill until required.**

Serving Suggestions: Serve chilled with a slice or two of fresh mango.

Storage: Will keep in the fridge for 2 days. Not suitable for freezing.

NUTRITIONAL ANALYSIS		Protein g	5.6	Fat g	0.6	Sodium g	0
PER PORTION		Carbohydrate g	22.4	Of which saturates g	0.3	Salt g	0
Energy kcal	110	Of which sugars g	16.6	Fibre g	0	Portion fruit and veg	1

Melon with Stem Ginger

Serves: 1   **Prep:** 5 minutes

55kcal and 0.3g fat per portion

Desserts have never been easier. Spice up melon with ginger in syrup. It adds a delicious kick.

150g cantaloupe
  melon
10g piece stem
  ginger in syrup
Mint leaves

1. Cut the melon into cubes and place in a serving bowl.
2. Finely chop the ginger and sprinkle over the top.
3. Decorate with mint leaves.

Serving Suggestions: Add a few raspberries or use 1 tbsp of cassis instead of the ginger.

Storage: Best served at once.

NUTRITIONAL ANALYSIS PER PORTION							
	Protein g	0.8	Fat g	0.3	Sodium mg		Trace
	Carbohydrate g	12.5	Of which saturates g	0	Salt g		Trace
Energy kcal 55	Of which sugars g	12.2	Fibre g	1.8	Portion fruit and veg		1

No-Fat Eton Mess

Serves: 2   **Prep:** 5 minutes
145kcal and 0.4g Fat per portion

Usually made with double cream and boasting a day's saturates per portion, this version of Eton Mess is almost fat free, and provides you with more calcium than cream would, too!

36g (3) meringue nests

100g fresh raspberries

100g fresh strawberries

150g fat-free Greek yogurt

150g virtually fat-free fromage frais

1. **Place the meringues in a plastic bag and give them a good bash to break them up, though do not crush them entirely.**
2. **Hull the fruit and halve the strawberries.**
3. **Mix together the yogurt and fromage frais in a large bowl, and stir in the fruit and meringues.**
4. **Spoon into 2 serving dishes and serve at once, or chill until required.**

Serving Suggestions: Eat at once!

Storage: Best eaten within a couple of hours of making, as the meringue becomes soggy otherwise.

NUTRITIONAL ANALYSIS PER PORTION		Protein g	13.1	Fat g	0.4	Sodium g	Trace
		Carbohydrate g	22.0	Of which saturates g	0.2	Salt g	Trace
Energy kcal	145	Of which sugars g	22.0	Fibre g	1	Portion fruit and veg	1

Oranges with Fresh Dates and Honey Yogurt

Serves: 1　**Prep:** 5 minutes

128kcal and 0.2g fat per portion

A simple tasty dessert that uses fresh dates. If they are not in season or you don't care for them, simply sprinkle over a handful of raisins instead.

1 medium (160g) orange

1 large fresh date (25g)

1 tbsp fat-free Greek yogurt

1 tsp runny honey

1. Cut the orange into segments over a bowl to catch any juice.

2. Pit and roughly chop the date and sprinkle over the orange segments.

3. Spoon over the yogurt and, lastly, drizzle over the honey.

Serving Suggestions: Eat at once!

Storage: As oranges are a great source of vitamin C, which is destroyed when exposed to the air, this is best not stored.

NUTRITIONAL ANALYSIS PER PORTION		Protein g	3.9	Fat g	0.2	Sodium mg	34
		Carbohydrate g	29.3	Of which saturates g	0	Salt g	Trace
Energy kcal	128	Of which sugars g	29.2	Fibre g	4.1	Portion fruit and veg	1

Pear and Chocolate Pudding

Serves: 4 or 6   **Prep:** 5 minutes   **Cook:** 30 minutes
290kcal and 4.5g fat ¼ per portion; 190kcal and 3g fat per ⅙ portion

A hot dessert that is easy to make and remarkably low in fat.

Oil-mister
2 medium eggs
110g caster sugar
120g plain flour
20g cocoa powder
240g canned pears in
   juice, drained

1. **Preheat oven to 200°C/180°C Fan/GM6 and lightly spray a shallow ovenproof dish measuring about 20cm diameter with oil.**
2. **Place the eggs and sugar in a bowl, and whisk with an electric whisk until light and fluffy.**
3. **Sieve in the flour and cocoa, and carefully fold in.**
4. **Pour the mixture into the prepared dish and arrange the pear halves on top.**
5. **Bake for 25–30 minutes until the sponge is springy and risen.**
6. **Remove from the oven and allow to cool for a few minutes before serving.**

Serving Suggestions: Serve with Bitter Chocolate Sauce (see page 252) or a scoop of low-fat vanilla ice cream.

Storage: Not suitable for storage.

Serves 4

NUTRITIONAL ANALYSIS PER PORTION		Protein g	7.8	Fat g	4.5	Sodium g	0.1
		Carbohydrate g	53.8	Of which saturates g	1.5	Salt g	0.2
Energy kcal	290	Of which sugars g	32.7	Fibre g	1.8	Portion fruit and veg	½

Serves 6

NUTRITIONAL ANALYSIS PER PORTION		Protein g	5.1	Fat g	3	Sodium g	0.1
		Carbohydrate g	35.5	Of which saturates g	1.0	Salt g	0.2
Energy kcal	190	Of which sugars g	21.6	Fibre g	1.2	Portion fruit and veg	½

Passion Fruit Crème Caramel

Serves: 4   **Prep:** 10 minutes   **Cook:** 45 minutes

128kcal and 4.1g fat per portion

Passion fruit is a wonderful addition to this classic dish. This version uses 1% fat milk, but you can use skimmed milk if you prefer, which will lower the fat content.

Oil-mister

50g sugar

575ml water

300ml 1% fat milk

2 large or 4 small passion fruit

2 eggs

1. Preheat oven to 170°C/150°C Fan/GM4.
2. Lightly spray 4 ramekins with oil.
3. Make the caramel by placing the sugar and 75ml of the water in a heavy-based saucepan and bringing very slowly to the boil. Allow the syrup to bubble until caramel in colour, then pour into the ramekins.
4. Meanwhile, warm the milk gently.
5. Scoop out the seeds and juice from one of the passion fruit into a sieve and press through using a spoon to collect the juice.

NUTRITIONAL ANALYSIS		Protein g	6.4	Fat g	4.1	Sodium g	Trace
PER PORTION		Carbohydrate g	17.4	Of which saturates g	1.4	Salt g	Trace
Energy kcal	128	Of which sugars g	17.4	Fibre g	0.5	Portion fruit and veg	0

6. Whisk the eggs and pour in the passion fruit juice.
7. Stir in the warm milk and pour through a sieve into the ramekin dishes.
8. Place the ramekins in a deep baking tray and pour in the remaining 500ml water to surround the ramekins.
9. Place in the oven for 45 minutes until the egg is set.
10. Remove from the oven and chill.
11. To serve, turn the puddings out into a bowl and scoop out the seeds and juice from the remaining passion fruit over the puddings.

Serving Suggestions: Serve with 80g fruit per person, such as strawberries, raspberries or chopped oranges. Made with semi-skimmed milk: 133kcal and 4.7g fat. Made with skimmed milk: 123kcal and 3.5g fat.

Storage: If covered, this will keep in the fridge for 2 days.

Pears with Lemon Grass and Coconut Sauce

Serves: 4   **Prep:** 10 minutes   **Cook:** 30 minutes

175kcal and 4.3g fat per portion

Pears poached in perry and lemon grass take on a different dimension, and the sauce, made by boiling down the poaching syrup and adding a tiny amount of coconut, really complements the fruit.

800g (4 medium)
Comice pears

500ml perry or dry cider

30g caster sugar

1 lemon grass stalk

25g creamed coconut

1 tsp cornflour or arrowroot

1 tbsp water

1. Peel the pears and place in a saucepan.
2. Pour the perry or cider over the pears and add the sugar and lemon grass.
3. Cover and gently poach for 30 minutes on top of the stove, or in a preheated oven at 160°C/140°C Fan/GM3 for 40 minutes.
4. Remove the pears from the syrup.
5. Boil the syrup down to achieve 300ml, then stir in the creamed coconut.
6. Stabilize the sauce with 1 teaspoon of cornflour or arrowroot mixed with 1 tablespoon water, cooking until it comes to a light boil.
7. Serve the pears and sauce at room temperature.

Storage: Can be stored for up to 2 days in the fridge.

NUTRITIONAL ANALYSIS	Protein g	1	Fat g	4.3	Sodium g	Trace
PER PORTION	Carbohydrate g	27	Of which saturates g	3.7	Salt g	Trace
Energy kcal	175	Of which sugars g	27	Fibre g	3.6	Portion fruit and veg	1

Poached Rhubarb with Vanilla 'Cream'

Serves: 2 **Prep:** 5 minutes **Cook:** 15–20 minutes
140kcal and 2.2g fat per portion

Simple but delicious. Look out for new-season rhubarb in May, which will be sweet and tender. The 'cream' is made from very low-fat soft cheese mixed with fat-free plain yogurt, which gives it a lovely smooth feel.

200g young rhubarb,
  cut into 7-cm pieces
25g caster sugar
2 tbsp water

For the vanilla 'cream'
Seeds from a vanilla
  pod or 1 tsp vanilla
  extract
100g extra-light soft
  cheese
100g fat-free plain
  yogurt
1 tsp icing sugar

1. Preheat oven to 190°C/170°C Fan/GM5.
2. Place the rhubarb in an ovenproof dish and sprinkle over the sugar, half the amount of vanilla and the water.
3. Cover and bake for 15–20 minutes until the rhubarb is tender. Remove from the oven and allow to cool.
4. Meanwhile mix together the soft cheese and yogurt along with the rest of the vanilla and the icing sugar. Chill until you are ready to serve.
5. To serve, spoon the rhubarb into a bowl along with the poaching liquid and place a spoon of the vanilla 'cream' next to it.

Serving Suggestions: Blitz the lot in a blender to make a fool – just chill afterwards.

Storage: Both items can be stored individually for 2 days in the fridge. The poached rhubarb can be frozen.

NUTRITIONAL ANALYSIS	Protein g	10.5	Fat g	2.2	Sodium g	0.2
PER PORTION	Carbohydrate g	18.8	Of which saturates g	1.3	Salt g	0.5
Energy kcal	140	Of which sugars g	18.7	Fibre g	1.4	Portion fruit and veg	1

Raspberry Oat Cranachan

Serves: 4   **Prep:** 15 minutes   **Cook:** 5 minutes

240kcal and 6.9g fat per portion

A Scottish favourite using some of Scotland's finest produce: raspberries, oatcakes and whisky.

50g plain oatcakes

50g jumbo porridge oats

25g muscovado sugar

20g butter

300g fat-free Greek yogurt

25ml whisky

25g runny honey

200g raspberries

1. Crush the oat cakes or place them in a food processor.
2. Mix together the oatcake crumbs, jumbo oats and sugar.
3. Melt the butter in a non-stick frying pan and add the crumb mixture. Gently cook over a low heat for 4–5 minutes, then allow to cool.
4. Mix together the yogurt, whisky and honey.
5. In individual tall glasses, place some raspberries at the base followed by the yogurt mixture and then some crumbs. Repeat, finishing with the crumb mixture. Chill until ready to serve.

Serving Suggestions: A glass of whisky would be perfect! Just add 88kcal for a 40ml tot.

Storage: Can be stored for 1 day in the fridge. Not suitable for freezing.

NUTRITIONAL ANALYSIS							
PER PORTION		Protein g	10.1	Fat g	6.9	Sodium g	0.1
		Carbohydrate g	34.3	Of which saturates g	3.5	Salt g	0.2
Energy kcal	240	Of which sugars g	18.6	Fibre g	1.5	Portion fruit and veg	½

Rice Pudding with Cardamom and Maple Syrup

Serves: 4   **Prep:** 2 minutes   **Cook:** 45 minutes

140kcal and 2g fat per portion

One of the most homely desserts, which you can cook in the oven or on the hob. This pudding is simply sweetened with maple syrup and is scented with cardamom seeds.

750ml 1% fat milk

60g pudding rice

5 cardamom pods, crushed

25g (1 tbsp) maple syrup

1. **Place all the ingredients in a non-stick saucepan and gently bring to simmering point.**

2. **Continue to simmer for 45 minutes until the rice is tender. Cool.**

3. **If more convenient you can cook this in an ovenproof dish for 45 minutes–1 hour at 170°C/150°C Fan/GM4.**

Serving Suggestions: Serve with a few blueberries or raspberries. Made with semi-skimmed milk: 150kcal and 3.2g fat. Made with skimmed milk: 125kcal and 0.6g fat.

Storage: Will keep in the fridge overnight, but is not suitable for freezing.

NUTRITIONAL ANALYSIS PER PORTION		Protein g	6.7	Fat g	2	Sodium g	Trace
		Carbohydrate g	23.8	Of which saturates g	1.0	Salt g	Trace
Energy kcal	140	Of which sugars g	12.2	Fibre g	0.4	Portion fruit and veg	0

Apple and Sultana Strudel

Serves: 4   **Prep:** 15 minutes   **Cook:** 30–40 minutes
200kcal and 3.7g fat per portion

Often loaded with butter and sugar, strudel can be a heavy treat. This one, however, uses only a little oil and minimum sugar, which helps you include it in your diet. If you don't have an oil spray, you can use a pastry brush.

25g (1 small slice) white bread, made into breadcrumbs

400g eating apples, such as Cox, peeled and cored

50g sultanas

Grated zest of 1 orange

15g demerara sugar

½ tsp mixed spice

96g (8 sheets) filo pastry

1 tbsp olive oil or oil spray

1 tsp icing sugar

1. Preheat oven to 190°C/170°C Fan/GM5.
2. Place the breadcrumbs on a baking sheet and allow to dry out in the oven for 5 minutes.
3. Grate or chop the apple and mix in a bowl with the sultanas, orange zest, sugar and spice.
4. Cut a large piece of foil and spray with a little oil.
5. Place a piece of filo on the foil and spray with oil. Repeat using all the pieces of filo, placing them on top of each other, but turning slightly each time, to make a large rectangular shape.
6. Place the breadcrumbs in the centre of the pastry and spoon the fruit mixture down the middle. Using the foil to help, roll up the strudel like a large sausage, tucking under the ends to prevent the filling from falling out.
7. Lightly spray the rolled-up strudel and bake for 30–40 minutes until lightly browned.
8. Cool and sieve with icing sugar.

Serving Suggestions: Serve with coffee after your meal.

Storage: Can be stored for 2–3 days in the fridge in an airtight container. Not suitable for freezing.

NUTRITIONAL ANALYSIS		Protein g	3.4	Fat g	3.7	Sodium g	0.2
PER PORTION		Carbohydrate g	40.7	Of which saturates g	0.5	Salt g	0.5
Energy kcal	200	Of which sugars g	26.9	Fibre g	3.0	Portion fruit and veg	1

Bites

Apricot and Coconut Muffins

Serves: 12 muffins   **Prep:** 10 minutes   **Cook:** 20 minutes

120kcal and 3.6g fat per muffin

These moist muffins make a great little dessert if you fancy something sweet without piling on the calories. Make a batch and freeze them so you can defrost one when you want it, rather than being tempted to eat too many at once.

400g can apricots in juice, drained

2 medium eggs

100g soft brown sugar

50g desiccated coconut

150g plain flour, sieved with 2 level tsp baking powder

1. **Preheat oven to 200°C/180°C Fan/GM6 and place 12 paper cases in a cake tray.**
2. **Drain the apricots and chop into small pieces, then place in a sieve and drain again.**
3. **Whisk the eggs and sugar together until light and fluffy using an electric whisk.**
4. **Fold in the coconut. Mix the flour and baking powder together and add to the egg mixture.**
5. **Lastly, carefully add the apricots.**
6. **Place in the oven for 20 minutes until risen and the cakes spring back when lightly pressed.**
7. **Cool on a wire rack.**

Serving Suggestions: Great with a cup of coffee for a simple dessert.

Storage: Store for up to 2 days in an airtight container. Can be frozen.

NUTRITIONAL ANALYSIS		Protein g	2.5	Fat g	3.6	Sodium g	Trace
PER PORTION		Carbohydrate g	20.3	Of which saturates g	2.5	Salt g	Trace
Energy kcal	120	Of which sugars g	10.8	Fibre g	1.0	Portion fruit and veg	0

Sundried Tomato and Black Olive Scones

Serves: 8   **Prep:** 10 minutes   **Cook:** 15 minutes
150kcal and 4.4g fat per scone

Delicious as a savoury snack or for lunch with soup, these scones will freeze or keep for a day or two in the fridge.

150g plain flour

100g wholemeal flour

2 level tsp baking powder

80g sundried tomatoes in oil, drained and chopped

100g black olives in brine, chopped

10g basil leaves

250g buttermilk

Black pepper

1. Preheat oven to 200°C/180°C Fan/GM6, and place a non-stick baking sheet on a baking tray.

2. Sieve together the flours and baking powder, adding the bran, which will collect in the bottom.

3. Mix in the tomatoes, olives, basil and buttermilk, and grind over some black pepper.

4. Make a soft but not sticky dough and place on a floured board.

5. Using a scone cutter, cut into 8 scones and place immediately on the baking sheet.

6. Place in the oven for 12–15 minutes until the scones are risen and browned.

7. Serve warm.

Serving Suggestions: Spread with low-fat soft cheese.

Storage: Will store in the fridge in an airtight container for 2 days. Warm through before serving. Suitable for freezing.

NUTRITIONAL ANALYSIS PER PORTION		Protein g	4.9	Fat g	4.4	Sodium g	0.3
		Carbohydrate g	24.6	Of which saturates g	0.4	Salt g	0.8
Energy kcal	150	Of which sugars g	2.1	Fibre g	2.1	Portion fruit and veg	0

Chocolate and Cheerios Fruit Snack

Serves: 12 small squares **Prep:** 10 minutes
80kcal and 2.8g fat per square

Breakfast cereals are usually very low in fat but fortified with useful vitamins and minerals. This snack may help satisfy any chocolate cravings you have, while keeping you within your targets. Just don't be tempted to eat too many!

100g milk chocolate

20g sweetened dried
  cranberries

50g sultanas

80g oat Cheerios

1. Melt the chocolate in a large bowl over a pan of simmering water.
2. Once it has melted, remove the bowl from the heat and stir in the dried fruits, followed by the cereal.
3. Press into an 18- to 20-cm square baking tin, and place in the fridge to set.
4. When it has set, cut into 12 pieces.

Serving Suggestions: Pop a piece in a small plastic bag to have with your coffee at work.

Storage: Keep in an airtight container in the fridge.

NUTRITIONAL ANALYSIS PER PORTION		Protein g	1.3	Fat g	2.8	Sodium g	0
		Carbohydrate g	12.6	Of which saturates g	1.5	Salt g	0
Energy kcal	80	Of which sugars g	9.4	Fibre g	0.	Portion fruit and veg	0

Chocolate Mallow Crispies

Serves: 12   **Prep:** 5 minutes   **Cook:** 5 minutes

100kcal and 2g fat per piece

A yummy chocolatey snack that fits into your calorie and fat target! Think about sharing them with your family and friends so you aren't tempted to eat more than you should!

100g milk chocolate, broken into small pieces

200g marshmallows

1 tsp vanilla essence

100g Rice Krispies cereal

1. Melt the chocolate in a large bowl over a pan of simmering water.
2. Add the marshmallows when the chocolate is runny, and keep stirring until the marshmallows have also melted completely.
3. Remove from the heat and stir in the vanilla and cereal.
4. Press into a baking tin about 20cm square. Chill.
5. When cool, remove from the fridge and cut into 16 pieces.

Serving Suggestions: With a glass of skimmed milk or cup of tea, this makes a tasty snack.

Storage: This will keep in an airtight container, preferably refrigerated, for 3–4 days. Not suitable for freezing.

NUTRITIONAL ANALYSIS		Protein g	1.4	Fat g	2	Sodium g	Trace
PER PORTION		Carbohydrate g	19.8	Of which saturates g	1.2	Salt g	Trace
Energy kcal	100	Of which sugars g	12.3	Fibre g	0.1	Portion fruit and veg	0

Maple and Raisin Drop Scones

Serves: 8 scones   **Prep:** 5 minutes   **Cook:** 10 minutes
85kcal and 2.8g fat per scone

Simple to make, these scones will keep for a day or two in the fridge and make a great snack or breakfast.

100g self-raising
  flour
1 egg
Grated zest of
  1 lemon
½ tsp cinnamon
15g (1 tbsp) maple
  syrup
1 tbsp sunflower oil
100ml semi-skimmed
  milk
25g raisins
Oil-mister

1. In a food processor or blender whiz all the ingredients together except the raisins to make a smooth pouring batter. Stir in the raisins.
2. Heat a non-stick frying pan and spray lightly with oil.
3. Use a tablespoon to pour 2–3 scones into the pan. Heat gently on one side, turning once, until lightly browned.
4. Repeat until all the batter is used up – the mixture should make about 8 scones.

Serving Suggestions: Serve with low-fat cheese or spread and a cup of tea. For 2 drop scones with a scraping (5g) of low-fat (40%) spread: 190kcal and 7.6g fat.

Storage: Store in an airtight container for 2 days. Can also be frozen.

NUTRITIONAL ANALYSIS PER PORTION		Protein g	2.5	Fat g	2.8	Sodium g	0.1
		Carbohydrate g	12.2	Of which saturates g	0.6	Salt g	0.2
Energy kcal	85	Of which sugars g	3.8	Fibre g	0.4	Portion fruit and veg	0

Mincemeat and Plum Filo Pies

Serves: 6   **Prep:** 10 minutes   **Cook:** 15–20 minutes
160kcal and 3.2g fat per pie

Adding plums to mincemeat adds moisture and flavour. This is a recipe that calls for an oil-mister, as it is quick and minimizes your use of oil.

150g mincemeat

250g plums,
   quartered and
   stones removed

125g filo pastry
   (about 10 small
   sheets)

Oil-mister

1. **Preheat oven to 190°C/170°C Fan/GM5.**

2. **Mix the mincemeat and plums together in a bowl.**

3. **Spray 1 sheet of pastry with a little oil and lay another on top of it at a 90-degree angle. Spray this lightly with oil, too, and place a spoon of the mincemeat and plum mixture in the centre.**

4. **Either roll up the pastry like a parcel, tucking the ends in, or draw up into a little pouch. Spray again very lightly.**

5. **Place on a baking sheet and repeat with the remaining pastry and mixture.**

6. **Bake for 15–20 minutes until the filling is cooked and the pastry a pale golden brown.**

7. **Cool.**

Serving Suggestions: Serve with reduced-fat ice cream or plain yogurt for a tasty dessert.

Storage: Keep in an airtight container for 3–4 days.

NUTRITIONAL ANALYSIS		Protein g	2.8	Fat g	3.2	Sodium g	0.1
PER PORTION		Carbohydrate g	29.4	Of which saturates g	0.8	Salt g	0.2
Energy kcal	160	Of which sugars g	18.5	Fibre g	0.7	Portion fruit and veg	¾

Orange and Sour Cherry Muffins

Serves: 12   **Prep:** 5 minutes   **Cook:** 20 minutes
160kcal and 2.7g fat per muffin

A fruity muffin that fits within your snack target; so make a batch to freeze and enjoy one when you have an urge for something sweet, happy in the knowledge that you are keeping within your limits.

50g olive spread or similar 60% fat

150g soft brown sugar

225g plain flour

3 level tsp baking powder

75ml freshly squeezed orange juice

Grated zest of 1 orange

2 tbsp skimmed milk

100g dried sour cherries

1. Preheat oven to 190°C/170°C Fan/GM5, and place 12 small muffin cases in a muffin tray.
2. Place all the ingredients except the cherries in a mixing bowl and mix with an electric mixer until smooth.
3. Stir in the cherries.
4. Spoon the mixture into the paper cases and bake for 18–20 minutes or until the cakes are risen and spring back when gently pressed.
5. Cool on a wire rack or cooling tray.

Serving Suggestions: Great with a cup of tea.

Storage: Will keep for 2–3 days in an airtight container. Are also suitable for freezing.

NUTRITIONAL ANALYSIS PER PORTION							
Energy kcal		160	Protein g	2.1	Fat g	2.7	Sodium g	Trace
			Carbohydrate g	34.8	Of which saturates g	0.6	Salt g	Trace
			Of which sugars g	19.6	Fibre g	1.0	Portion fruit and veg	0

Spelt and Walnut Scone Round

Serves: 8 **Prep:** 10 minutes **Cook:** 15–20 minutes
200kcal and 8g fat per piece

Spelt is an ancient grain, which has recently been revived in the UK. It provides a nutty flavour and texture that you can, if you prefer, replace with wholemeal flour. Scones make a great addition to breakfast as well as teatime meals.

120g plain white flour
3 level tsp baking powder
130g spelt (or wholemeal) flour
25g olive oil spread
25g sugar
60g walnuts, roughly chopped
150ml semi-skimmed milk

1. Preheat oven to 200°C/180°C Fan/GM6 and lightly spray a baking sheet with oil.
2. Sieve the white flour and baking powder into a mixing bowl and add the spelt or wholemeal flour.
3. Rub the olive spread into the flour, then add the sugar and walnuts.
4. Use a blunt knife to stir the milk into the dry ingredients to make a moist but not sticky dough.
5. Sprinkle a little flour on a chopping board or clean work surface, and shape and lightly roll the dough into a 20-cm round.
6. With a sharp knife score into 8 segments, then bake for 15–20 minutes until the scone is lightly browned.
7. Cool then serve, split or cut into the 8 pieces.

Serving Suggestions: 1 portion spread with very low-fat (20%fat) spread and 1 tsp (5g) jam: 245kcal and 9.3g fat.

Storage: Will keep for a couple of days in an airtight container, but also freezes very well.

NUTRITIONAL ANALYSIS		Protein g	5.4	Fat g	8	Sodium mg	Trace
PER PORTION		Carbohydrate g	16.6	Of which saturates g	1.2	Salt g	Trace
Energy kcal	200	Of which sugars g	4.8	Fibre g	2.3	Portion fruit and veg	0

Orange Bran Loaf

Serves: 8 slices   **Prep:** 10 minutes + 1 hour soak   **Cook:** 45 minutes
210kcal and 2.1g fat per slice

This is like breakfast all at once – bran flakes, orange juice, raisins and eggs, all combined to make a delicious, simple loaf that you can enjoy for breakfast, lunch or tea!

100g raisins

50g bran flakes

300ml unsweetened
  orange juice

2 eggs

50g soft brown
  sugar

225g plain flour

3 level tsp baking
  powder

1. Place the raisins and bran flakes in a bowl and pour over the orange juice. Leave for a minimum of 1 hour or until the bran flakes are softened.

2. Preheat oven to 190°C/170°C Fan/GM5 and line a large (10-cm x 15-cm) loaf tin with baking parchment.

3. Beat the eggs and sugar together in a large bowl and stir in the softened bran flakes, juice and raisins.

4. Sieve the flour and baking powder together and stir into the mixture.

5. Pour the mixture into the prepared tin and bake for 40–45 minutes until the loaf springs back when gently pressed.

6. Remove from the oven and allow to cool for 5 minutes before turning out.

7. Cool and store in an airtight container for up to 3 days.

Serving Suggestions: Enjoy for breakfast with a cup of tea, coffee or juice. Alternatively, enjoy as a snack.

Storage: Store in the fridge in an airtight container for up to 3 days.

NUTRITIONAL ANALYSIS		Protein g	5.7	Fat g	2.1	Sodium g	Trace
PER PORTION		Carbohydrate g	44.7	Of which saturates g	0.5	Salt g	Trace
Energy kcal	210	Of which sugars g	19.5	Fibre g	2.0	Portion fruit and veg	½

Cheese and Apple Scones

Serves: 10   **Prep:** 10 minutes   **Cook:** 15 minutes

165kcal and 5.9g fat per scone

These moist cheesey scones will liven up your lunchbox or breakfast. Use mature cheddar to minimize fat and maximize taste.

225g plain flour
50g wholemeal flour
3 level tsp baking powder
50g olive spread or other fat containing 60% fat
200g cooking apples, peeled, cored and roughly chopped
75g mature cheddar, grated
160ml skimmed milk, plus a little for brushing

1. Preheat oven to 220°C/200°C Fan/GM7, and place a non-stick baking sheet on a baking tray.
2. Sieve the flours and baking powder into a large bowl, adding back the bran (which will remain in the sieve).
3. Rub in the spread and then add the cooking apples and half the cheese.
4. Stir in the milk to make a soft but not sticky dough.
5. Place the dough on a lightly floured board and roll to about 1.5-cm thickness. Using a 6-cm cutter, cut out 10 scones and place on the baking sheet.
6. Brush the scone tops with a little milk and sprinkle over the remaining cheese.
7. Bake for 15 minutes or until the scones are golden brown and risen.

Serving Suggestions: Serve with soup at lunchtime, or for a delicious breakfast.

Storage: Will keep for 2 days in an airtight container. Suitable for freezing.

NUTRITIONAL ANALYSIS		Protein g	5.3	Fat g	5.9	Sodium g	Trace
PER PORTION		Carbohydrate g	23.5	Of which saturates g	2.4	Salt g	Trace
Energy kcal	165	Of which sugars g	3	Fibre g	1.5	Portion fruit and veg	0

Recipes by kcal per portion

Breakfasts and Brunches

Ham and Cheese Toastie	380
Scrambled Egg on Toast	337
Poached Egg Muffin with Spinach and Mushrooms	300
Greek Yogurt with Berries and Walnuts	295
Smoked Salmon with Baby Dill Pancakes	290
Four-grain Porridge with Apricots	260
Grapefruit Salad with Toasted Almonds	220
Breakfast Compote	205
Breakfast Smoothie	160
Buttermilk Pancakes	95
Piquant Egg and Watercress Sandwich	365
Bacon- and Sweetcorn-stuffed Sweet Potato	335
Mozzarella and Ham Panini	315
Bruschetta with Mozzarella, Basil and Tomatoes	310
Ciabatta Roll with Pesto, Soft Cheese and Baby Spinach	310
Smoked Trout Sandwich with Horseradish and Lamb's Lettuce	310
Hot Prawn Tortilla Wrap	305
Chicken Tikka Pitta with Raita	235
Roasted Pepper and Halloumi Panini with Watercress and Clementine Salad	141

Soups

Bacon and Sweetcorn Chowder	320
Moroccan Chickpea and Fruit Soup	185
Pea Soup with Pesto Croute	170
Curried Parsnip and Apple Soup	140
Cauliflower and Almond Soup	125
Chinese-style Soup with Tiny Pork Balls	112
Creamy Cherry Tomato Soup	111
Watercress Soup	110
Pumpkin Soup	105
Carrot and Celery Soup	70

Sandwiches and Light Lunches

Turkey and Mango Mini-naan	450
Baked Potato with Ratatouille and Goats Cheese	405
Ham and Caramelized Red Onion Chutney	390
Tuna and Sweetcorn Bagel (Dairy-free)	390
Warm Wrap with Refried Beans, Avocado and Peppers	380
Baked Potato with Curried Prawns	375

Main Course Salads

Pasta, Pesto and Chicken Salad	440
Tuna and Black Olive Bulghar Wheat Salad	410
Tuna and Edamame Salad with Avocado and Green Beans	395
Pear and Feta Salad	390
Summer Salad with Ciabatta	375
Smoked Mackerel with Carrot and Currant Salad	360
Asparagus and Egg Salad with Baby New Potatoes	330
Hot Garlicky King Prawn Salad	300
Red Grape and Edam Salad	277
Pearl Barley and Pomegranate Salad	175

Poultry

Chicken, Fennel and Soya Bean Fricassée	507
Apricot Chicken with Almonds and Pearl Barley	485
Duck with Water Chestnuts and Noodles	455

Chicken Masala with Yogurt and Rice	441
Turkey and Leek Risotto	435
Oriental Mushrooms and Turkey with Rice Noodles	410
Coronation-style Turkey with Fresh Mango	400
Chicken with Cherry Tomato and Leek Mash	382
Turkey Burgers with Tomato and Red Onion Salad	335
Mexican Chicken in Chocolate	330
Chicken and Peanut Stir-fry	314
Baked Chicken and Peaches with Lime and Sour Cream	306
Greek Baked Chicken with Okra	305
Coq au Vin	275
Chicken with Cajun Spices and Chickpeas	265
Sunflower Seed-coated Chicken with Yogurt Herb Salad	250
Chicken Fillets with Dill and Sundried Tomatoes	234
Chicken and Parma Parcels	228
Turkey Steaks with Crumb and Sundried Tomato Topping	222
Minty Chicken with Leek	190

Meat

Pork and Butternut Squash Cumberland Pie	508
Jambalaya	500
Pork Tenderloin Stuffed with Apple and Cranberry	485
Old-fashioned Steak and Kidney Cobbler	453
Pork in Dijon Mustard Sauce with Leek Mash	445
Beef in Beer with Mustard Mash	405
Fresh Pea and Ham Risotto	400
Steak and Mangetout Stir-fry	370
Home-made Burgers with Spicy Potato Wedges	360
Lamb and Apricot Tagine	380
Lamb and Coconut with Noodles	335
Marinated Lamb with Crushed Potatoes	335
Moussaka	326
Beef Koftas with Tzatziki	325
Steak with Sage and Red Wine Sauce	320
Pork Chop in Citrus Sauce	323
Chilli con Carne	315
Topside with Winter Vegetables	315
Venison with Plums and Port	315
Gammon with Sweet-and-sour Shallots	310
Spicy Lamb	302
Pork with Lime and Wine Sauce	300
Maple Lamb with Butternut Squash	292
Beef with Sweet Chestnuts	275
Pork with Plums and Chinese Spices	265
Ragu	240
Pork Patties	205
Skewered Pork and Mango	205
Grilled Teriyaki Pork with Orange	176

Fish and Seafood

Cherry Tomato and Smoked Haddock Kedgeree	450
Scallop and Prawn Chow Mein	422
Italian Tuna with Black Olives and Tomatoes	420
Seafood Paella	416
Lemony Salmon with Thyme Couscous and Onion Salad	410
Special Fish Pie	400
Tandoori Fish with Spicy Okra	400
Plaice and Parma Ham Rolls with Roasted Vegetables	365
Pickled Herring with Beetroot Slaw	360
Bacon-wrapped Pollack with Baked Cherry Tomatoes	350
Trout Fillet with Crushed Peas	308
Smoked Haddock Fish Cakes	306
Prawns with Sweet Potato and Lime	305

Mediterranean Fish in Filo Parcels	270
Simple Cod Bake	260
Baked Plaice with Warm Lentil Salad	217
Polenta-crusted Cod with Tarragon Sauce	210
Monkfish and Prawn Kebabs	202
Seabass with Lemon Grass and Baby Corn	190
Sundried Tomato-topped Seafood Bake	180

Vegetarian

Tricolour Risotto	450
Mushroom Stroganoff with Rice	430
Galettes with Spinach, Mushroom and Soft Goat's Cheese	320
Chipotle Lentils	295
Stuffed Butternut Squash	290
Pepperonata with Baked Eggs	250
Mushroom and Feta Filo Pouches	235
Courgette and Celery Filo Pie	216
Lentil and Spinach Dhal with Cardamom	210
Three bean curry	200

Sides

Citrus Couscous	248
Apricot and Ginger Rice	200
Leek and Mustard Mash	185
Coconut Rice	170
Polenta with Parmesan and Shallots	165
Boulangère Potatoes	150
Potatoes with Mustard Seeds and Spinach	146
Sweet Potato and Swede Mash	142
Beetroot Slaw	138
Crushed New Potatoes with Herbs and Olive Oil	135
Okra with Tomatoes	128
Warm Potato Salad with Herbs	120
Watercress and Orange Salad	115

Greek Peas with Leek and Mint	95
Braised Red Cabbage	85
Ratatouille	85

Pasta

Baked Rigatoni with Celery, Ham and Cider	500
Lasagne	500
Salmon and Asparagus Linguine	500
Fusilli with Red Pepper and Olive Sauce	465
Spaghetti with Chilli Prawns	450
Butternut Squash and Bacon with Wholemeal Spaghetti	445
Spinach and Mushroom Pasta Bake	410
Tripoline with Lemon Mushrooms	400
Pasta Sauce with Artichokes and Peppers	106
Pasta Sauce with Mediterranean Vegetables	88

Sauces, Dressings and Dips

Smoked Trout Paté	125
Home-made Houmous	123
Bitter Chocolate Sauce	70
Pomegranate Sauce	60
Blueberry and Orange Coulis	50
Pineapple Salsa	46
Chive Dip	36
Raspberry Salsa	33
Spicy Harissa Dressing	30
Sweetcorn Salsa	30
Chilli and Coriander Dressing	29
Apple and Mint Dressing	27
Raita	23
Fat-free Yogurt and Herb Dressing	16
Tomato and Coriander Salsa	13

Desserts

Poached Rhubarb with Vanilla 'Cream'	240
Apple and Cranberry Crisp	238
Apple and Sultana Strudel	200

Pear and Chocolate Pudding	190
Pears with Lemon Grass and Coconut Sauce	175
Baked Plums with Port	158
Baked Peaches with Amaretti Filling	155
No-fat Eton Mess	145
Raspberry Oat Cranachan	140
Rice Pudding with Cardamom and Maple Syrup	138
Oranges with Fresh Dates and Honey Yogurt	128
Passion Fruit Crème Caramel	128
Summer Fruit Compote	125
Bramley and Mango Brûlée	120
Mango and Kiwi Salad with Blackcurrant Sorbet	117
Mango Fool	110
Autumn Fruit Salad	100

Melon with Stem Ginger	55
Fruits of the Forest Mousse	50
Fruits of the Forest Soufflé	50

Bites

Orange Bran Loaf	210
Spelt and Walnut Scone Round	200
Cheese and Apple Scones	165
Mincemeat and Plum Filo Pies	160
Orange and Sour Cherry Muffins	160
Sundried Tomato and Black Olive Scones	150
Apricot and Coconut Muffins	120
Chocolate Mallow Crispies	100
Maple and Raisin Drop Scones	85
Chocolate and Cheerios Fruit Snack	80

Recipes by Fat per portion

Breakfasts and Brunches

Greek Yogurt with Berries and Walnuts	13.9
Poached Egg Muffin with Spinach and Mushrooms	12.8
Scrambled Egg on Toast	11.7
Ham and Cheese Toastie	11.6
Grapefruit Salad with Toasted Almonds	11.5
Smoked Salmon with Baby Dill Pancakes	10.8
Buttermilk Pancakes	3
Four-grain Porridge with Apricots	3
Breakfast Smoothie	1.8
Breakfast Compote	0.4

Soups

Bacon and Sweetcorn Chowder	13.2
Creamy Cherry Tomato Soup	6.3
Pea Soup with Pesto Croute	5.5
Curried Parsnip and Apple Soup	5.4
Pumpkin Soup	4.9
Watercress Soup	4.7
Cauliflower and Almond Soup	4.5
Moroccan Chickpea and Fruit Soup	4.3
Chinese-style Soup with Tiny Pork Balls	3.2
Carrot and Celery Soup	1.7

Sandwiches and Light Lunches

Mozzarella and Ham Panini	15.6
Bacon- and Sweetcorn-stuffed Sweet Potato	14.6
Warm Wrap with Refried Beans, Avocado and Peppers	13.8
Roasted Pepper and Halloumi Panini with Watercress and Clementine Salad	13.2
Ciabatta Roll with Pesto, Soft Cheese and Baby Spinach	12.2
Piquant Egg and Watercress Sandwich	11.3

Baked Potato with Ratatouille and Goats Cheese	10.9
Bruschetta with Mozzarella, Basil and Tomatoes	10.8
Baked Potato with Curried Prawns	8.5
Turkey and Mango Mini-naan	8.3
Smoked Trout Sandwich with Horseradish and Lamb's Lettuce	7.7
Ham and Caramelized Red Onion Chutney	7.6
Hot Prawn Tortilla Wrap	7.1
Tuna and Sweetcorn Bagel (Dairy-free)	6.2
Chicken Tikka Pitta with Raita	3.6

Main Course Salads

Summer Salad with Ciabatta	15.2
Tuna and Edamame Salad with Avocado and Green Beans	15.1
Asparagus and Egg Salad with Baby New Potatoes	14.8
Smoked Mackerel with Carrot and Currant Salad	14.6
Red Grape and Edam Salad	13.4
Pasta, Pesto and Chicken Salad	12
Pear and Feta Salad	11.5
Tuna and Black Olive Bulghar Wheat Salad	8.5
Hot Garlicky King Prawn Salad	8.2
Pearl Barley and Pomegranate Salad	3.6

Poultry

Greek Baked Chicken with Okra	15.3
Chicken and Peanut Stir-fry	14.9
Chicken Masala with Yogurt and Rice	14.3
Coq au Vin	13.5
Apricot Chicken with Almonds and Pearl Barley	12.9
Baked Chicken and Peaches with Lime and Sour Cream	12.4
Chicken, Fennel and Soya Bean Fricassée	12.4

Turkey Burgers with Tomato and Red Onion Salad	11.8
Chicken Fillets with Dill and Sundried Tomatoes	11.3
Coronation-style Turkey with Fresh Mango	10
Turkey and Leek Risotto	9.4
Duck with Water Chestnuts and Noodles	9.2
Chicken with Cherry Tomato Reduction and Leek Mash	9.1
Chicken with Cajun Spices and Chickpeas	7.7
Oriental Mushrooms and Turkey with Rice Noodles	6.9
Sunflower Seed-coated Chicken with Yogurt Herb Salad	6.5
Chicken and Parma Parcels	6.1
Turkey Steaks with Crumb and Sundried Tomato Topping	6.1
Mexican Chicken in Chocolate	6
Minty Chicken with Leek	4.9

Meat

Old-fashioned Steak and Kidney Cobbler	15.6
Moussaka	14.8
Beef Koftas with Tzatziki	14.3
Pork and Butternut Squash Cumberland Pie	14.1
Spicy Lamb	13.9
Pork in Dijon Mustard Sauce with Leek Mash	12.7
Chilli con Carne	12.6
Home-made Burgers with Spicy Potato Wedges	12.1
Gammon with Sweet-and-sour Shallots	12
Steak with Sage and Red Wine Sauce	11.9
Marinated Lamb with Crushed Potatoes	11.8
Pork Tenderloin Stuffed with Apple and Cranberry	11.8
Jambalaya	11.4
Lamb and Apricot Tagine	11.2

Pork Chop in Citrus Sauce	10.9	Polenta-crusted Cod with	
Pork Patties	10.9	Tarragon Sauce	5.1
Beef with Sweet Chestnuts	10.5	Seabass with Lemon Grass and	
Maple Lamb with Butternut		Baby Corn	5.1
Squash	10.4	Baked Plaice with Warm Lentil	
Steak and Mangetout Stir-fry	9.3	Salad	3.8
Fresh Pea and Ham Risotto	9.2		
Ragu	8.7	**Vegetarian**	
Lamb and Coconut with		Stuffed Butternut Squash	13.6
Noodles	8.2	Mushroom Stroganoff with Rice	13.4
Beef in Beer with Mustard Mash	8.1	Pepperonata with Baked Eggs	13.4
Topside with Winter Vegetables	7.8	Galettes with Spinach,	
Pork with Plums and Chinese		Mushroom and Soft Goat's	
Spices	6.8	Cheese	12.5
Pork with Lime and Wine Sauce	5.6	Courgette and Celery Filo Pie	12.3
Skewered Pork and Mango	5.4	Tricolour Risotto	11.3
Grilled Teriyaki Pork with Orange	4.2	Chipotle Lentils	11.2
Venison with Plums and Port	3.2	Mushroom and Feta Filo	
		Pouches	9.8
Fish and Seafood		Lentil and Spinach Dhal with	
Lemony Salmon with Thyme		Cardamom	4.5
Couscous and Onion Salad	15.3	Three bean curry	4.5
Trout Fillet with Crushed Peas	14.1		
Pickled Herring with Beetroot		**Sides**	
Slaw	13.6	Potatoes with Mustard Seeds	
Mediterranean Fish in Filo		and Spinach	5.6
Parcels	13.4	Polenta with Parmesan and	
Cherry Tomato and Smoked		Shallots	4.8
Haddock Kedgeree	12.8	Coconut Rice	4.5
Bacon-wrapped Pollack with		Greek Peas with Leek and Mint	4.4
Baked Cherry Tomatoes	12.3	Warm Potato Salad with Herbs	3.8
Italian Tuna with Black Olives		Apricot and Ginger Rice	3.7
and Tomatoes	12.2	Okra with Tomatoes	3.7
Plaice and Parma Ham Rolls		Crushed New Potatoes with	
with Roasted Vegetables	12.2	Herbs and Olive Oil	3.5
Tandoori Fish with Spicy Okra	11	Boulangère Potatoes	3.4
Scallop and Prawn Chow Mein	10.2	Leek and Mustard Mash	1.5
Smoked Haddock Fish Cakes	9.5	Sweet Potato and Swede Mash	1.3
Prawns with Sweet Potato and		Ratatouille	1.2
Lime	9	Watercress and Orange Salad	0.6
Simple Cod Bake	8.7	Braised Red Cabbage	0.5
Special Fish Pie	8.2	Citrus Couscous	0.2
Monkfish and Prawn Kebabs	7.7	Beetroot Slaw	0.4
Sundried Tomato-topped			
Seafood Bake	6.5		
Seafood Paella	6		

Pasta

Butternut Squash and Bacon with Wholemeal Spaghetti	15
Lasagne	14.4
Salmon and Asparagus Linguine	13.3
Spaghetti with Chilli Prawns	13
Fusilli with Red Pepper and Olive Sauce	12.4
Spinach and Mushroom Pasta Bake	11.7
Tripoline with Lemon Mushrooms	8
Baked Rigatoni with Celery, Ham and Cider	7.6
Pasta Sauce with Artichokes and Peppers	6.9
Pasta Sauce with Mediterranean Vegetables	4.8

Sauces, Dressings and Dips

Home-made Houmous	7.3
Smoked Trout Paté	4.9
Spicy Harissa Dressing	2.8
Bitter Chocolate Sauce	2.4
Chive Dip	2.1
Pomegranate Sauce	1
Raspberry Salsa	0.3
Sweetcorn Salsa	0.3
Pineapple Salsa	0.2
Tomato and Coriander Salsa	0.2
Blueberry and Orange Coulis	0.1
Chilli and Coriander Dressing	0.1
Fat-free Yogurt and Herb Dressing	0.1
Raita	0.1
Apple and Mint Dressing	0

Desserts

Apple and Cranberry Crisp	7.9
Poached Rhubarb with Vanilla 'Cream'	6.9
Pears with Lemon Grass and Coconut Sauce	4.3
Passion Fruit Crème Caramel	4.1
Apple and Sultana Strudel	3.7
Pear and Chocolate Pudding	3
Raspberry Oat Cranachan	2.2
Rice Pudding with Cardamom and Maple Syrup	2
Baked Peaches with Amaretti Filling	1.3
Mango Fool	0.6
Summer Fruit Compote	0.5
Mango and Kiwi Salad with Blackcurrant Sorbet	0.4
No-fat Eton Mess	0.4
Autumn Fruit Salad	0.3
Melon with Stem Ginger	0.3
Baked Plums with Port	0.2
Bramley and Mango Brûlée	0.2
Oranges with Fresh Dates and Honey Yogurt	0.2
Fruits of the Forest Mousse	0.1
Fruits of the Forest Soufflé	0.1

Bites

Spelt and Walnut Scone Round	8
Cheese and Apple Scones	5.9
Sundried Tomato and Black Olive Scones	4.4
Apricot and Coconut Muffins	3.6
Mincemeat and Plum Filo Pies	3.2
Chocolate and Cheerios Fruit Snack	2.8
Maple and Raisin Drop Scones	2.8
Orange and Sour Cherry Muffins	2.7
Orange Bran Loaf	2.1
Chocolate Mallow Crispies	2

Chapter 5

Eating Out

In recent years the number of meals that we eat away from the home has increased markedly, whether it's a quick sandwich when out shopping, a coffee and muffin on the way to work or a more formal occasion in a restaurant. This trend reflects the busy on-the-go lifestyle that many of us lead, too busy to prepare food or even to sit down to eat it. Couple this with the lack of time or motivation to be active in our leisure time, and no wonder we see levels of obesity rising.

Eating out in a restaurant should be an enjoyable experience, but when you are trying to lose weight it is sometimes a source of anxiety. This chapter contains helpful tips for when you are eating out and about. It covers a range of cuisines so that you can make wise choices and avoid picking the fattiest meal on the menu.

It can also be hard to know which sandwiches or salads are suitable to eat when you are following a diet. This chapter provides nutrition information on a range of different shop-bought lunch choices to help you choose one that fits in with your diet.

The old adage 'the best intentions can be dissolved in alcohol' has some truth in it when trying to keep to a diet. Your plan to have one glass of wine while you wait for your meal can easily sabotage your efforts when the food is late and the waiter tops you up. Alcohol, though fat-free, is high in calories and may weaken your resolve, so energy values for alcohol are also provided in this chapter.

Help with Menus and Tips for When You Dine Out

Read this section when you are planning to go out for a meal so that you can enjoy yourself without over-indulging or feeling miserable and deprived because you don't know what to choose.

- Eat normally during the day rather than 'saving up' calories and fat for a blow-out. If you do this you are much more likely to exceed your fat target, and may be so hungry you find it difficult not to overeat. In fact, having a small snack such as a glass of skimmed milk, a banana or a few plain breadsticks before you go out will take the edge off your appetite so you can choose from the menu without being disturbed by the sound of your tummy rumbling.
- While you are choosing from the menu, have a glass of water, whether fizzy or plain, rather than an alcoholic drink, saving this for when the food comes. Also avoid eating more than 1 small piece of bread while you are waiting for your food. If you are tempted to demolish a basket of bread, just say you don't want bread, or ask your fellow diners to keep it out of reach!
- Do ask for help with the menu if you are unclear how a food is cooked, or you have some specific requests. Ask the waiter for his or her recommendations for someone following a reduced-fat diet. Or you may simply want to request:
  - that any sauces are served separately rather than poured over your food
  - a smaller portion of a main course
  - that any salad dressing or oil is served separately, so you can choose whether and how much to add
  - that hot vegetables are not glazed with butter
  - that your food (e.g. steak, chops, some fish) is grilled rather than fried
  - a sorbet or fresh fruit for dessert

What Does It Mean?

Some restaurants like to write some or all of their menus using terms that can be difficult to understand. The terms, which are often French or Italian, are a guide to the way in which the food is cooked or which ingredients they contain. Knowing this can help you avoid the high-fat ones and choose those that are more suitable when you are trying to lose weight. Below is a list of some terms and dishes you may come across.

Term	Meaning or content	Tactic in the restaurant
Fermière	Meat or poultry cooked with vegetables. Tends not to be high in fat	OK
À la grecque	As in 'Greek' – containing herbs, lemon juice and olive oil	Find out how much oil is added to the dish
Dauphinois	Cooked in cream and garlic	Avoid – have plain potatoes
Florentine	Cooked with spinach, and sometimes a creamy sauce	Ask about the sauce, then decide
Lyonnaise	Usually cooked with buttery onions, vinegar and parsley	Limit or avoid
Marinière	Fish or shellfish such as mussels cooked in white wine	OK
Meunière	Usually fish dipped in flour then fried in butter	Avoid. Ask for grilled fish
À la milanaise	Usually a food that is egg-, cheese- and crumb-coated then fried	Avoid
Niçoise	Often a salad with green beans, eggs, tuna, olives and tomatoes	OK in small amounts Ask for separate dressing
À la Normande	Could contain cider, apples, cream, butter	Find out more; if very creamy avoid, if just apples and cider go ahead
À la Provençale	Contains Mediterranean vegetables such as tomatoes, peppers, garlic	Usually OK but ask how much olive oil is used
Alfredo	Usually a pasta sauce made with cream, butter and parmesan	Avoid – try a tomato-based sauce instead
Alla arrabiata	A tomato- and chilli-based pasta sauce	OK

Alla cacciatora	Usually meat or poultry braised with tomatoes, herbs and mushrooms	OK
Alla giardino	Usually cooked with garden vegetables	Check whether creamy or oily
Au beurre	Cooked with butter	Avoid
Au gratin	Cooked with a crust of breadcrumbs and cheese, so can be high in fat	Avoid or ask about how much cheese and fat it contains
Au jus	Usually applied to meat served in its own cooking juices	OK
Beignet	Deep-fried pastries	Avoid
Béarnaise sauce	A rich sauce based on hollandaise sauce	Avoid
Bisque	A creamy seafood soup	Avoid – try a lighter soup or consommé
Chasseur	Poultry or game cooked in red wine sauce with mushrooms	OK in medium portions
Crème brûlée	A rich egg-and-cream dessert topped with caramelized sugar	Avoid
Crème caramel	A light egg-and-milk dessert with caramel, often made with skimmed milk	OK
En brochette	Cooked on a skewer and grilled	OK
En croûte	Cooked in a parcel of rich pastry	Avoid
En papillote	Cooked in a parcel of paper or foil	OK
Flambé	Food that is covered in spirit and lit. Tends to be higher-fat foods such as pancakes.	Find out more then decide
Fricassée	Chicken cooked in a rich, creamy sauce	Avoid
Fritto misto	A mixture of deep-fried foods	Avoid
Hollandaise sauce	A rich egg-and-butter sauce	Avoid
Mornay sauce	A creamy sauce enriched with egg yolks and Gruyère cheese	Avoid
Panna cotta	A rich creamy dessert	Avoid
Pâté	These usually are high in fat. Vegetable pâtés are often based on cheese	Avoid

Friday Night's All Right to Diet

In this section you will find some tips to help you make sensible diet choices in a range of different types of restaurants. The best advice is always to ask about the food: how it is prepared and cooked.

Indian or Other Asian Restaurants

Spicy and delicious but often high in fat from the ghee, oil or coconut, much Asian food is not great when you are dieting. However, there are safer options, and some foods of which a small portion is fine.

Good choices include foods that are cooked in a tandoori oven, or grilled without heavy sauces. Try tandoori or tikka dishes (not tikka masala), and chicken or prawn jalfrezi or dopiaza. Dishes that are cooked in cream, coconut or almonds are off-limits. These include korma, pasanda and masalas.

While you are waiting for your meal don't indulge in poppadums, which are deep fried, and if you have pickles, stick to those that are low in fat.

Choose plain rice rather than pilau or biryani and, if you like to have bread, make this an alternative to rice and go for plain chapati rather than naan breads.

Chinese

As with other restaurants, Chinese cuisine can present a lot of diet pitfalls, so go prepared to change your regular order for something different.

Many main-course dishes are deep fried, or battered *and* deep fried, so avoid these! This includes prawn crackers, which look innocent but are not! Choose simple stir-fries, asking if minimal fat can be added. Vegetable dishes tend to be lower in fat than meat, duck or poultry, and are best eaten with plain rice rather than egg-fried varieties.

Similarly, avoid the prawn toast or spring roll starters, which are high in fat and calories, opting for clear soups instead. Obviously fatty meats such as spare ribs and duck are best avoided, and if you fancy chicken or pork just ask how it is cooked, and if it is fried then steer clear. Foods that are steamed, such as dumplings, are usually lower in fat – but may be quite calorific. Steamed fish or poultry and vegetables are perfect.

Italian

There is a lot more to Italian cuisine than pizza and pasta, which is good news when you are on a diet, as pizza tends to be high in calories and fat, and pasta is very energy-dense, making a small portion higher in calories than you may expect.

Good options when eating Italian are seafood or grilled poultry, with an undressed side salad, and if you have pasta, choose a light tomato-based sauce rather than a creamy or cheese-based one. Garlic bread is loaded with butter, so give it a miss, but if everyone else is indulging ask for bread sticks, which you can nibble (slowly) to keep them company. Italian puddings such as panna cotta and tiramisu are going to be off your menu, but you can have fresh fruit in season: some delicious strawberries, fresh figs, or perhaps some caramelized oranges, or enjoy a light sorbet or granita.

Spanish or Mexican

They share a language and historical roots, so no wonder the cuisine has similarities.

Mexican-style restaurants tend to be big on filled items such as tacos, tortillas and enchiladas, which can be fried as well as filled with high-fat ingredients. So approach with caution, asking lots of questions, and opt for plain tortillas with bean or vegetable fillings without added cream, cheeses or avocados. Burritos, which are usually smaller and steamed, are a good choice if the filling is low-fat.

A salsa or sauce in Mexican cuisine is usually tomato based or at least lower in fat than guacamole or sour cream, so should be OK with some grilled fish or chicken.

Tapas dishes in Spanish restaurants can vary enormously, so do ask what each contains and go for those that seem to have the highest proportion of vegetables and potatoes to meat or fish and those that haven't been fried. Also ask for the dish not to be covered in olive oil.

Recipes of course vary from place to place, so the best policy is to find out how a dish is prepared. The spicy, cold tomato soup gazpacho, for example, can be low in fat when olive oil is not used in the recipe, but quite high when it is. However, white garlic soup (ajo blanco) always uses lots of almonds, so give this one a miss.

Seafood is often a good option: try clams and mussels in broth or oven-baked white fish in tomato or vegetable sauces, which don't feature too much oil or cream.

Grilled fish, meat and poultry with plain cooked vegetables or salad are a safe option whatever the restaurant, and it need not be boring especially when cooked with flavoursome herbs, lemon and wine.

Greek

The Greeks, like the Spanish and Italians, have an innate love of olive oil, and this abounds in many of the dishes you will find in a Greek restaurant. Armed with this knowledge you should ask for olive oil to be served separately so the choice to add it remains with you.

Grilled poultry and fish, or lean kebabs, provided they are not doused with oil before cooking (ask) and eaten with plain salad and pitta bread, make a good diet choice. One dish that is usually heavy in oil and therefore should be avoided is moussaka, and this goes for pastichio as well.

Seafood, whether shellfish or fish steaks or fillets, is a good choice especially if simply cooked without added oil.

The content of a Greek salad can vary enormously, so choose this if it has mostly tomatoes, cucumber, lettuce and onions, with limited feta cheese and olives. Again, ask for it to come without olive oil.

Houmous, taramasalata and falafel are tasty starters but usually too high in fat for dieters. Stuffed vine leaves (dolmades) may be a better option.

French

With one of the most highly developed and regarded international cuisines, it can be difficult to generalize about French cuisine, but mention of cuisine minceur may give the restaurateur a guide to what you are looking for.

The section 'What Does It Mean?' (see page 294) may be your best guide when eating in a French restaurant.

Choose a light starter such as a consommé, fruit or salad without dressing and avoid pâtés, terrines and thick creamy (velouté) type soups.

Opt for a small portion of grilled white fish or chicken, with a light sauce with plain or boulangère potatoes rather than creamy gratin Dauphinois or any frites.

Try to find out whether fresh seasonal fruit is served, and choose this instead of a rich dessert or the tempting array of cheeses.

Pub Meals

Traditional British pub cuisine, where you still find it, can be difficult for a dieter. So choose carefully, opting for meat (not cheese) ploughman's lunches, and jacket potatoes with baked beans rather than butter and cheese. Give pasties of any sort a miss, as pastry is high in fat and calories.

Soup and a sandwich may be fine if the soup isn't creamy and the sandwich has a low-fat filling. Ask for it to be made without mayonnaise and using no or minimal butter or spread, and ask for extra salad on the side instead of crisps.

Traditional main meals such as shepherd's pie or fish pie can be eaten in small portions, with plenty of vegetables, but watch out for steak-and-kidney pudding and pies, which can be high in fat and calories. Look for stews or casseroles served with vegetables and boiled potatoes, rather than chips or roast potatoes.

Pizza

Pizzas can be tricky for dieters, as most are high in fat and calories. If the restaurant is part of a chain, find out if there is nutrition information on their website, and use this to guide you. The best diet advice is not to go to pizza outlets unless you are prepared to compromise and eat only a small amount. If this is OK for you then choose a thin crust with vegetable toppings, lean ham or prawns, and no or minimal amounts of cheese. Toppings such as jalapeños and olives in brine can be used in moderation, but avoid pepperoni, sausage, extra cheese and fried vegetables, and especially cheese-stuffed crusts.

Don't be tempted to have side dishes such as coleslaw (which will be loaded with mayonnaise) or garlic bread. Keep it small and simple!

Burgers/Other Fast Food

Like pizza chains, some fast-food outlets provide nutrition information on their websites so you can peruse the menu in advance. However, most people go on impulse to these eateries, so here are some tips. Avoid anything that says 'fried' or 'crispy', as both are synonymous with fat. Choose small and plain with salad not cheese, with low-fat dressings not mayonnaise or creamy dressing. Not all food is off-limits in fast-food outlets; a few suitable choices are flagged up in the tables that follow.

Nutrition Information

Realistically, most of us don't make our own lunch every day, so included here are a range of different places where you may go and buy lunch. It should help you identify which ones fit your diet targets for calories and fat. The lists for sandwiches include rolls, wraps and 'subs'. There's also data on salads.

It is beyond the scope of this book to provide information on all possible retail outlets, so this has been restricted to retailers who responded to an invitation to provide data, and a few other outlets whose information is easily accessible through the internet. The information was correct at the time of going to press.

Sandwiches

Sandwiches can be high in fat from spreads, mayonnaise and cheesey fillings, so watch out when you are out. The ones listed here have been nutritionally analysed by the manufacturer, and picked for this book because they should fit with your diet.

Boots

Name of sandwich	per portion		
	kcal	Fat g	size g
Shapers			
Egg Mayonnaise & Cress	302	8	161
Salmon & Cucumber	305	5.2	187
Tuna & Cucumber	285	4.7	187
Prawn Mayonnaise	297	6.7	178
Chicken Salad	274	4.5	183
Coronation Chicken	312	4.2	176
Chicken No Mayo	310	4.4	175
Chicken & Bacon	324	7.1	193

Name of sandwich	per portion		
	kcal	fat g	size g
Mature Cheddar & Fruit Chutney	348	9	197
Shapers Flatbreads			
Falafel	264	4.6	198
Tex Mex Chicken and Salsa	267	5.8	187
Shapers Wraps			
Sweet Chilli Chicken Wrap	276	3.3	159
Barbecue Chicken Wrap	286	4	172
Red Thai Chicken Wrap	258	4	168
Houmous & Falafel Wrap	292	6.4	185
Prawn & Rocket Wrap	218	4.1	159

Marks & Spencer

Name of sandwich	per portion		
	kcal	fat g	size g
Count On Us			
Tuna and Red Pepper Crunch	275	2.7	unknown
3 Cheese and Celery	250	4.2	unknown
Ham Salad on Oatmeal Bread	260	5.8	unknown
Fuller Longer			
Deep Filled Roast British Chicken and Pesto Flatbread	310	10.2	unknown
Nacho Chicken Tortilla	300	4.6	unknown
Deep Filled Tandoori and Lentil Dhal Flatbread	310	5.2	unknown
Ham, Cheese and Mustard	320	7.5	unknown
Other Lines			
Just … Wild Red Salmon and Cucumber Sandwich	320	12.5	unknown
Just … British Ham on White	290	6.9	unknown
Just … Tuna and Sweetcorn	390	13.3	unknown
Classic – Tuna Crunch Submarine	360	10.7	unknown
Classic – British Roast Chicken and Salad	385	11.7	unknown
Classic – Prawn Cocktail	330	12.3	unknown
Crayfish and Rocket	380	12.8	unknown
Hoisin Duck Wrap	380	11.0	unknown

Pret A Manger

Name of sandwich	per portion		
	kcal	Fat g	size g
Scottish Smoked Salmon	348	11.5	158
Slim Pret – Beech Smoked BLT	248	14.4	124
Slim Pret – Chicken Avocado	232	12.4	122

Sainsbury's

Name of sandwich	per portion		
	kcal	Fat g	size g
Be Good to Yourself			
Humous and Crunchy Vegetable	342	7.8	unknown
Chicken Tikka less than 3% fat	296	3.4	unknown
Tuna & Cucumber less than 3% fat	293	4.9	unknown
Roast Chicken Salad less than 3% fat	273	3.8	unknown
Egg & Cress 30% less fat	268	7.5	unknown
Prawn Cocktail 30% less fat	280	8.1	unknown
Cheese Ploughman's 30% less fat	314	10.5	unknown
Honey & Mustard Chicken Salad	305	4.4	unknown

Subway

Name of sandwich	per portion		
	kcal	Fat g	size g
Low Fat			
Beef Sub with Salad	271	3.2	221
Ham Sub with Salad	258	3.7	221
Sweet Onion Chicken Teriyaki Sub with Salad	352	4.3	278
Turkey Breast and Ham with Salad	266	3.7	230
Chicken Breast with Salad	297	4	235
Subway Club	298	4.1	254
Turkey Breast Sub	256	3.2	221
Veggie Delight	202	1.8	164
Breakfast			
Bacon Sub	268	7.5	98
Sausage Sub	364	12.7	156
Bacon and Egg Sub	331	13.5	135

Starbucks

Name of sandwich	per portion		
	kcal	Fat g	size g
Lunch Panini			
Chicken and Pesto	349	8	unknown
Chicken Pastrami	411	12.8	unknown
Falafel	362	7.1	unknown
Toastie			
Mini Cheese and Ham	327	11.1	unknown
Sandwich			
Roast Chicken and Herb Mayo	325	7.3	unknown
Wrap			
Roast Chicken Salsa	364	8.3	unknown

Tesco

Name of sandwich	per portion		
	kcal	Fat g	size g
Chicken Salad	385	13.01	212
Hoisin Duck Wrap	337	8.46	184
Roast Chicken and Stuffing	456	15.76	197
Seafood Cocktail	376	15.98	170
Prawn and Egg	382	12.33	190
Roast Chicken	384	12.28	168

Waitrose

Name of sandwich	per portion		
	kcal	Fat g	size g
Spicy Jerk Chicken with Mango Salsa on Pepper & Chilli Bread	344	8.17	190
Chicken Fajita Wrap with Crunchy Lettuce, Fresh Coriander & Salsa	290	6.56	174
Tuna with Chunky Cucumber & Lemon Vinaigrette	251	5.27	195
Mixed Peppers, Houmous & Baby Spinach on Pepper & Chilli Bread	268	6.63	170
Egg Mayo with Crunchy Salad on Brown Bread with Bran & Poppy Seeds	302	10.11	206

Name of sandwich	per portion		
	kcal	Fat g	size g
Roast Chicken with Mixed Leaves, Juicy Vine Tomatoes			
& Mayonnaise	325	6.26	197
Prawn Cocktail with Cruncy Cucumber & Juicy Vine			
Tomatoes on Oatmeal Bread	300	8.09	196
Mediterranean Style Tuna with Crunchy Salad on Pepper			
& Chilli Bread	262	3.84	202
Spicy Chicken Tikka on Kolonji Seed Bread	354	9.8	190
Wiltshire Ham & Piccalilli with Mixed Leaves & Mayonnaise	343	6.15	201
Spicy King Prawn with Mango on Kolonji Seed Bread	302	8.6	180
Wrap Selection Sweet Chilli Chicken, Chicken Caesar,			
Hoisin Duck	281	9.39	139
Chicken & Mango Open Sandwich	247	8.1	137
Wild Crayfish with Lemon Mayo & Rocket	178	5.63	96
British Ham with English Mustard	323	9.21	151
Seafood Cocktail with Crunch Cucumber on Oatmeal Bread	328	8.14	203
Hoisin Duck Wrap with Crunchy Iceberg Lettuce			
& Spring Onions	317	9.9	155
Wiltshire Ham in White Bread	282	5.27	134

Salads

The word salad covers many foods that are served chilled, from mayonnaise-rich potato salad and coleslaw to fat-free watercress. Main course salads that provide a better balance of carbohydrates, fat and protein are shown here if they will fit within your diet.

Boots

Name of salad	per portion		
	kcal	Fat g	size g
Shapers Salads			
Chicken Caesar	174	6	188
Honey Mustard Chicken Pasta	328	7.3	252
Tuna & Sweetcorn Pasta	321	3.9	259
King Prawn Noodles	296	4.4	258

Name of salad	per portion		
	kcal	Fat g	size g
Three Bean	134	1.3	210
Greek Pasta	224	6.5	215
Chicken Fajita Chicken Pasta	316	6.2	271
Tuna Nicoise	130	3.5	219
Shapers Sushi			
Chicken	254	3.6	155
Veggie Selection	240	2.9	155
Fish Selection	268	6.4	159
Fish & Veg Selection	257	3.6	155

Marks & Spencer

Name of salad	per portion		
	kcal	Fat g	size g
Fuller Longer			
Tomato and Basil Chicken, Couscous & Squash	290	7.4	230
Count On Us			
Tuna Layer Salad	270	8.8	340
Vietnamese Chicken Salad	140	4.4	275

Pret a Manger

Name of salad	per portion		
	kcal	Fat g	size g
Deluxe Sushi	380	6.8	250
Vegetable Sushi	277	5.4	193

Sainsbury's

Name of salad	per portion		
	kcal	Fat g	size g
BGTY Orzo and Sunbaked Tomato	315	7.3	unknown
BGTY Caesar	141	8.1	unknown
BGTY Couscous with Chargrilled Vegetables	74	0.7	unknown

Waitrose

Name of salad	per portion		
	kcal	Fat g	size g
King Prawn Noodle	259	5.23	275
Smokey Mixed Bean	152	6.48	120
Chicken, Butterbean & Turmeric Rice	262	8.51	230
King Prawn Noodle	204	6	200
Fruity Moroccan Couscous	139	3.24	90
Tuna with Lemon and Caper Mayonnaise on Malted Bread	320	6.77	209
Greek Feta with Black Olives and Tzatziki	209	9.14	112
Tabbouleh	83	2.07	90

Going For a Drink?

It's amazingly easy to clock up calories on the most innocuous-looking drinks, whether they are alcoholic or not. So here is a selection of commonly consumed coffee-shop drinks to illustrate what they may contain. Just make sure that you count both the calories and fat in your daily allowance when you are out for a drink, and keep it below 3g fat when it is a snack. Don't forget that sugar adds calorie too. For each teaspoon of sugar you are adding 20kcal.

Coffee Shops

Starbucks

Name of drink	per portion		
	kcal	Fat g	size ml
Cappuccino			
Tall cappuccino, made with whole milk	108	5.6	354
Tall cappuccino, made with semi-skimmed milk	91	3.4	354
Tall cappuccino, made with soya	72	2.6	354
Tall cappuccino, made with skimmed milk	64	0.1	354
Latte			
Tall latte, made with whole milk	176	9.2	354
Tall latte, made with semi-skimmed milk	148	5.6	354
Tall latte, made with soya	116	4.3	354
Tall latte, made with skimmed milk	102	0.2	354

Name of drink	per portion		
	kcal	Fat g	size ml
Hot Chocolate with Whipped Cream			
Tall hot chocolate, made with whole milk	319	16.2	354
Tall hot chocolate, made with semi-skimmed milk	294	12.9	354
Tall hot chocolate, made with soya	265	11.8	354
Tall hot chocolate, made with skimmed milk	258	7.9	354

Costa

Name of drink	per portion		
	kcal	Fat g	size ml
Cappuccino			
Medio cappuccino, made with whole milk	101	4.7	Unknown
Medio cappuccino, made with soya	77	3.2	Unknown
Medio cappuccino, made with skimmed milk	58	0.2	Unknown
Latte			
Medio latte, made with whole milk	128	6.9	Unknown
Medio latte, made with soya	86	4	Unknown
Medio latte, made with skimmed milk	71	0.3	Unknown
Hot Chocolate with Whipped Cream and Marshmallows			
Medio hot chocolate, made with whole milk	321	15.5	Unknown
Medio hot chocolate, made with skimmed milk	294	11.0	Unknown

Pubs and Bars

Unwinding with a glass of wine or lager may be your regular start to the evening, but remember that the calories from alcohol are metabolized first by your body, before it starts to burn fat, so keep your alcohol consumption tightly limited, and preferably only drink with a meal.

Most alcoholic drinks are fat-free, with the exception of a few alcopops, and creamy liqueurs, but all supply calories. Alcohol provides more calories per gram than carbohydrate and protein and almost as much as fat.

Type of drink	Drink name	Serving	kcal
Alcopop	Breezers	275ml bottle	160–180
	Smirnoff ice or black ice	275ml bottle	176
	Red Square	275ml bottle	170–220
	WKD	275ml bottle	220–230
Beers	Draught mild	568ml (Pint)	136
	Average bitter	568ml (Pint)	170
	Average low-alcohol bitter	568ml (Pint)	75
	Average premium or best bitter	568ml (Pint)	185–190
Ciders	Average in low-alcohol	568ml (Pint)	95–100
	Average (sweet or dry)	568ml (Pint)	190–240
Lagers	Average regular	568ml (Pint)	185–230
	Average export	568ml (Pint)	210–250
	Average low-alcohol	568ml (Pint)	55–65
Wine	White, dry	175ml	116
	White, medium	175ml	130
	White, sparkling	175ml	130
	Rosé	175ml	124
	Red	175	119
	Vermouth, dry	50ml	54
	Vermouth, sweet	50ml	76
Spirits	Gin, vodka, whisky 37.5% proof	35ml	72
	Gin, vodka, whisky 40% proof	35ml	78

Chapter 6

Going Shopping

Understanding which foods are suitable for your diet will be crucial for you to succeed, so it is really important that you know how to interpret the information found on food labels. This chapter will help you to do just that so that you can shop confidently, knowing what you can put in your basket and what is best left out.

Also, knowing that there will be days when you don't fancy cooking or haven't the time, this chapter provides information on a wide range of ready meals from UK retailers that are suitable for your diet.

What's on the Label?

Although it is not compulsory, most foods sold in the UK provide some sort of nutrition labelling. This may be very simple, such as:

Cereal bar

	Per 100g
Energy	393kcal
Protein	8g
Fat	8g
Carbohydrate	73g

This label shows you that 100g of the product contains 8g of fat. However, it does not tell you how big the portion is, nor how many grams of saturated fat are in the 8g total. This type of simple nutrition labelling is common in other European countries. In the UK there will usually be a more detailed label:

Cereal bar

	Per 100g	Per bar (23g)
Energy	393kcal	90kcal
Protein	8g	2g
Carbohydrate	73g	17g
of which sugars	34g	17g
Fat	8g	2g
of which saturates	4g	0.9g
Fibre	2.5g	0.6g
Sodium	0.25g	0.05g
Salt equivalent	0.65g	0.1g

This label is really useful for dieters as you can see straight away that it has 2g of fat per bar and 90 calories (kcal). This means it would be OK to eat it as a snack, as it fits within the 3g fat and 150kcal maximum target. You would still, of course, need to make sure that it didn't take you over your daily total targets.

Other labelling schemes have also been developed in the UK over the last few years. One uses traffic lights to alert you to the overall healthfulness of foods. Another scheme shows how the food fits within your whole diet, by using reference points called Guideline Daily Amounts (GDAs).

Guideline Daily Amounts

GDAs are designed to help with choosing a healthier diet by providing information about a food and comparing it to the average amount of energy or nutrients that an average adult needs each day.

In the example opposite, the panel shows you that 180g of pizza provides 458 calories and 18.6g of fat. This means that it will be unsuitable for your diet (in this size portion) as it exceeds most calorie and fat targets. However, you could eat half (90g) as the amount of fat would then be 9.3g and the calories 229kcal.

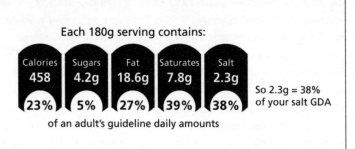

Each 180g serving contains:

Calories	Sugars	Fat	Saturates	Salt
458	4.2g	18.6g	7.8g	2.3g
23%	5%	27%	39%	38%

So 2.3g = 38% of your salt GDA

of an adult's guideline daily amounts

What the label also shows you is how much this portion provides of the energy, sugar, fat, saturates or salt recommended for an adult. The pizza provides 23% of the calories recommended for an adult not trying to lose weight. Whilst following this diet you have your own personal guideline daily amounts for fat and calories, so not all this information is relevant to you. However, in the long term this information can help you assess whether or not a food is suitable for inclusion in your regular diet.

Traffic Light Scheme

The other commonly used scheme in the UK is the Food Standards Agency's traffic light scheme.

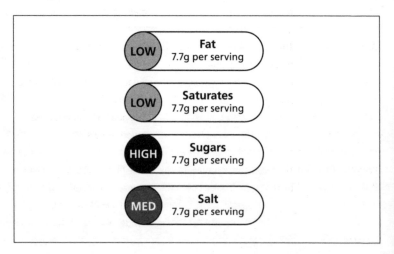

LOW — Fat 7.7g per serving

LOW — Saturates 7.7g per serving

HIGH — Sugars 7.7g per serving

MED — Salt 7.7g per serving

The traffic light scheme shows how much fat, saturates, sugars and salt are contained within one portion of the food. The colour then indicates whether this is considered to be low, medium or high, which suggests how readily you should eat this food. Green means go ahead as it is low in that nutrient, while red means that the food is high in something we need to cut down on, so the food should only be eaten occasionally. When a nutrient is amber the food is an OK choice most of the time, but other foods in your diet should be green for that nutrient. This scheme may help you with your overall choices when shopping, particularly when focusing on the fat you are permitted in your daily target.

Low-Fat or Reduced-Fat?

Often foods have labels that make claims about the fat content, and this can be very confusing. Manufacturers have to follow legislative guidelines including a recent European directive that has outlawed some commonly made but misleading claims; however, you may still find some foods with these claims on the supermarket shelves (because manufacturers are given a grace period in which to update their packaging).

Low-Fat	A food must contain less than 3g of fat for every 100g of food, in other words it contains 3% fat.	These foods are genuinely low fat and are useful when dieting. Choose some of these foods when on your diet.
Reduced-Fat	The term 'reduced-fat' means that the food contains 30% less fat than the equivalent standard version.	If the food is a high-fat food such as cheese or cream, it may still contain a lot of fat. Look for the number of fat grams per 100g and how much fat one portion contains.
Fat-Free	The food cannot contain more than 0.5g of fat per 100g.	These fat-free foods may be high in sugars, so be careful not to overindulge. Sugars still provide calories.

	This claim is no longer permitted as it is misleading. No products should have a '% fat-free' claim unless it is totally fat-free, when it can say 'fat-free' – see page 313.	You may find a few of these, or similar claims, such as 95% fat-free on the shelves, but these should not be there much longer. Check how many grams of fat one portion contains.
90% fat-free		
Lite or light	If this term is used it has to have 30% less fat than the equivalent standard version.	If the food is a high fat food, it may still contain a lot of fat. Look out for the number of fat grams per 100g and how much fat one portion contains.

Buying Ready Meals

There are times when you want to let someone else do the food preparation as you are too busy, tired or unmotivated. On these occasions a ready-prepared meal can be useful. Chosen wisely – checking that the fat and calorie content fits within your meal targets – they can be a real help.

In the tables that follow, some of the best-selling ready meals from the major supermarkets are shown, along with the fat and calorie content per portion. You can use these to make up your own meal plan, adding vegetables or starchy accompaniments as needed (look at Chapter 9 for nutrition information on these).

Major UK supermarkets were invited to send nutrition information for this book in Autumn 2008. The resulting tables use a selection of ready meals that fit the diet guidelines and were correct at the time of going to press.

The tables are sorted according to brand, range, and then by fat content.

Marks & Spencer

Name of Food	Pack weight	Portion weight	kcal	Fat g
Count On Us Range				
Spaghetti carbonara	365	365	385	8.0
Chicken tikka massala with rice	400	400	400	8.0
Creamy roasted mushroom risotto	375	375	340	5.6
Vegetable moussaka	400	400	280	10.8

Name of food	Pack weight	Portion weight	kcal	Fat g
Pasta magharita	360	360	360	8.3
Roasted cherry tomato risotto	360	360	340	6.1
Ricotta and spinach cannelloni	400	400	380	10.8
Chicken and tomato tagliatelle	400	400	360	5.7
Chargrilled chicken and asparagus risotto	385	385	325	6.5
Spaghetti and meatballs	400	400	340	6.4
Chicken jalfrezi and special basmati rice	400	400	400	6.8
Beef lasagne	365	365	365	10.2
Cajun chicken fettuccine	400	400	380	8.0
Risotto primavera with asparagus and peas	375	375	340	7.1
Tuna and pasta bake	400	400	400	8.4
Stonebaked mushroom and ham pizza	245	245	355	4.4
Stonebaked ham and pineapple pizza	230	230	370	3.7
Orkney crab and asparagus risotto	400	400	380	8.0
Chicken korma and special basmati rice	365	365	400	8.4
Mild vegetable curry and pilau	400	400	340	0.8
Chicken and vegetable chow mein	380	380	265	4.9
Steak and vegetable Yorkshires	320	160	200	3.2
Roast pork loin, new potatoes, carrots and cabbage	395	395	275	9.9
Sweet and sour chicken with rice	400	400	360	2.0
Lemon and ginger chicken with rice	400	400	400	6.4
Lamb and spring vegetable casserole	390	390	265	6.6
Fish pie with haddock, king prawns and salmon	400	400	260	7.2
Chicken breast with gravy mash, carrots and peas	400	400	300	5.2
Cottage pie	400	400	340	8.0
Fuller Longer Range				
Thai green curry with jasmine rice	400	400	400	10.0
Seafood linguine, king prawns, scallops and salmon	400	400	400	9.2
Roast beef meatballs and spaghetti	400	400	400	10.8
Ham hock, tangy mustard sauce, mash and veg	400	400	300	8.0
Beef and chianti ragu	400	400	440	14.4
Shepherd's pie	440	400	395	14.4
Steak and mushroom pie with luxury mash	440	440	410	9.0
Chicken and vegetable hotpot	420	420	380	7.6

Name of Food	Pack weight	Portion weight	kcal	Fat g
Chicken, roasted squash and edamame bean risotto	420	420	485	9.7
Hoisin duck with noodles	400	400	335	7.4
Singapore noodles, chicken and king prawns	400	400	380	12.0
3 mushroom tagliatelle with creamy sauce	370	370	445	13.0
Chicken tikka biryani and lentil pilau	400	400	480	10.0
Beef stroganoff and rice	400	400	400	8.8
Vegetarian Range				
Roast mushroom and caramelised onion pie	400	400	280	10.0
Filled pepper halves	295	147	135	5.2

Sainsbury's

Name of Food	Pack weight	Portion weight	kcal	Fat g
Be Good to Yourself Range				
BGTY less than 3% fat Beef in ale	–	–	295	5.4
BGTY less than 3% fat Cod mornay	–	–	282	5.3
BGTY Shepherd's pie reduced fat	–	–	314	9.4
BGTY less than 3% fat Vegetable curry	–	–	263	1.8
BGTY less than 3% fat Thai green chicken curry	–	–	354	5.2
BGTY less than 3% fat Ham & roasted mushroom tagliatelle	–	–	399	8.5
BGTY less than 3% fat Mediterranean vegetable pasta	–	–	413	5.4
BGTY Fish pie reduced fat	–	–	392	12.2
BGTY less than 3% fat Chilli jacket potato	–	–	318	6.3
BGTY less than 3% fat Cajun chicken pizza	–	–	425	6
BGTY less than 3% fat Spinach & ricotta pizza	–	–	424	5.6
BGTY less than 3% fat King prawn masala	–	–	410	6.8
BGTY Cottage pie reduced fat	–	–	334	8.8
BGTY Chicken & mushroom pie reduced fat	–	–	356	11.9
BGTY less than 3% fat Tomato & basil chicken with roasted baby potatoes	–	–	315	6.8
BGTY less than 3% fat Spaghetti bolognese	–	–	405	9.1
BGTY reduced fat Penne bolognese bake	–	–	471	10.3
BGTY less than 3% fat Prawn primavera	–	–	383	6.1

Name of Food	Pack weight	Portion weight	kcal	Fat g
BGTY less than 3% fat Cauliflower cheese	–	–	93	3.2
BGTY Mushroom risotto reduced fat	–	–	387	8.7
BGTY less than 3% fat Chilli con carne	–	–	381	8.7
BGTY reduced fat Macaroni cheese	–	–	484	10
BGTY reduced fat Spinach & ricotta cannelloni	–	–	366	11.3
BGTY less than 3% fat Vegetable lasagne	–	–	339	7.9
BGTY less than 3% fat Chicken chow mein	–	–	361	9.2
BGTY less than 3% fat Singapore noodles	–	–	317	9.9
BGTY less than 3% fat Sweet & sour chicken	–	–	423	4.3
BGTY less than 3% fat Chicken jalfrezi	–	–	406	5.1
BGTY less than 3% fat Chicken arrabbiata	–	–	412	6
BGTY less than 3% fat Chicken tikka masala	–	–	429	7.6
BGTY less than 3% fat Chicken korma	–	–	376	5.4
BGTY reduced fat Beef lasagne	–	–	383	9.4
BGTY less than 3% fat Sausage & mash	–	–	338	9.8
BGTY less than 3% fat Paprika chicken & rice	–	–	393	6.6
Be Good to Yourself Frozen Range				
BGTY less than 3% fat Bolognese pasta bake	–	–	306	5.4
BGTY less than 3% fat Chicken and mushroom risotto	–	–	306	5
BGTY less than 3% fat Chicken tikka masala with rice	–	–	373	5.2

Tesco

Name of Food	Pack weight	Portion weight	kcal	Fat g
Light Choices				
Chicken chow mein	400	400	420	7.5
Chicken pasta bake	400	400	429	6.4
Sweet and sour chicken with rice	400	400	405	1.5
Chicken tikka with rice	450	450	470	7.1
Lamb moussaka	350	350	230	7.4
Spaghetti bolognaise	400	400	420	8.8
Cottage pie	450	450	372	11
Cheese and broccoli pasta	350	350	431	8
Chicken in peppercorn sauce	400	400	413	3.6

Name of Food	Pack weight	Portion weight	kcal	Fat g
Lasagne	400	400	392	9.6
Beef enchiladas	400	400	386	8.3
Beef in red wine with colcannon mash	400	400	284	7.6
Chicken hot pot	360	360	251	4.2
Chicken and broccoli pie	450	450	318	8.7
Chicken and gravy pie	450	450	350	7.4
Chilli con carne and rice	500	500	486	7.5
Spaghetti carbonara	400	400	468	8.4
Spaghetti and meatballs	400	400	404	10.4
Spicy beef pasta	350	350	480	5.1
Spinach and ricotta pasta	350	350	439	12.3

Waitrose

Name of Food	Pack weight	Portion weight	kcal	Fat g
Low Saturated Fat				
Chilli con carne with rice	400	400	421	4.8
Mushroom risotto	400	400	402	9.6
Green Thai chicken curry with jasmine rice	370	370	441	8.51
Macaroni cheese	370	370	449	7.77
Prawn linguine	400	400	387	10.8
Chicken and asparagus with roast potatoes	400	400	408	10.8
Moussaka	350	350	303	10.85
Cottage pie	400	400	313	6
Chicken jalfrezi with pilau rice	400	400	395	6
Ham and mushroom tagliatelle	400	400	445	10
Chicken with madeira wine & porcini mushrooms	415	415	378	11.21
Lasagne	400	400	388	10.4
Fisherman's pie	399	399	300	7.2
Chicken korma with pilau rice	395	395	399	3.95
Chicken tikka masala with pilau rice	400	400	416	5.2
Chicken saag with pilau rice	400	400	378	4
Beef stroganoff with rice	400	400	429	6.4

Name of Food	Pack weight	Portion weight	kcal	Fat g
Deliciously Different				
King prawn and scallop paella with black rice, peppers and spinach	360	360	354	7.45
Halloumi cheese with a warm salad of beans and lentils in a tomato dressing	399	399	360	12.8
Salmon tagliatelle with petits pois, asparagus and fresh spinach	355	355	338	7.46
Salmon, king prawns & scallops in a fresh tomato sauce with wholewheat spaghetti	370	370	367	9.73
Lentil & edamame bean salad with goat's cheese	330	330	374	13.2
King prawn Thai salad with wild rice & sugar snaps	325	325	337	3.9
Pearl barley and seafood risotto with yellow cherry tomatoes, salmon, king prawns & crab	375	375	331	7.13
Thai green chicken curry with Thai fragrant rice, water chestnuts, sugar snaps & pak choi	350	350	441	10.15
Chicken and prawn jambalaya with brown rice, chargrilled peppers and sweet potato	390	390	388	14.04
Slow cooked BBQ beef with chargrilled sweet potato, peppers and spicy pinto bean sauce	380	380	306	8.36
Chermoula chicken with Israeli couscous and a lightly spiced yoghurt dressing	350	350	420	14
Core				
Asparagus & babycorn masala	150	150	111	6.75
Beef goulash	300	300	278	9.51
Liver & bacon with mashed potato	399	399	331	9.2
Cauliflower cheese	225	225	164	10.8
Steak & ale meal for one	399	399	359	11.6

Chapter 7

Exercise

Managing our weight is a balance of the calories we consume and the calories we use. If you eat more calories than your body needs, those extra calories automatically get stored as fat, resulting in you putting on unnecessary weight. The best way for you to combat this and use up those excess calories is to get more physically active in your daily lifestyle. This is often much harder than just reducing the calories you consume.

Making physical activity part of your lifestyle will ensure that you achieve your goals quicker, and will make maintaining your weight more manageable.

Exercise is so important to the human body, especially now that so many of us lead such sedentary lifestyles. We now live in a convenience society where everything is available at the touch of a button or with very little effort. This can have very detrimental effects on people's health, both physical and mental. So what can we do? Well, there are thousands of people who fit some kind of physical activity into their lives. Health clubs and leisure centres can now be found almost anywhere, offering a variety of different activities for you to do and enjoy. However, exercise does not have to be as structured as this; a half-hour walk at lunchtime would be sufficient and goes a long way to improving your health.

Later in the chapter we will illustrate just how you can do exercise just about anywhere and anytime! First, let's take a look at some of the many reasons why you should do your best to get some regular exercise.

Why Exercise?

Strengthening Your Circulatory and Cardiovascular System

As your heart and lungs strengthen you will find doing everyday tasks easier. This will in turn make it easier to lead an active lifestyle.

Weight Management

Increased activity levels help your body burn more calories, resulting in weight loss and helping you to keep your weight under control.

Combating Illness

As well as boosting your immune system, preventing you from catching some colds or the flu, exercise can also help to prevent some chronic diseases such as heart and lung diseases and even cancer. It will lower blood pressure and help to reduce cholesterol, leaving your body much stronger and ready for action. (Published by BUPA's health information team, August 2007.)

Feeling Great

Exercise releases chemicals into your body, which leave you feeling happier and more relaxed. Exercising at the right time can help you to relax especially at the end of a busy day. The after-effects of improved fitness, weight loss and tone will help you feel great about yourself.

Lower Stress Levels

Lowering stress levels is very important in today's society, and getting more exercise will help with this. Exercising is such a positive thing to do for yourself, and as your body starts to change shape and feel great you will start to feel better about yourself and the things going on around you.

Improved Social Life

Exercise does not have to be done alone, in fact more and more people now seek to train with partners, friends and in groups for extra motivation and support. Lots of people make new friends in the gyms and classes or wherever they do their exercise, finding people with the same exercise goals as themselves.

Types of Exercise

'Exercise' is one word for an endless amount of activities that can be performed by the human body, from abseiling and wall-climbing to gym-based programmes, dance classes or just kicking a ball around with your children. Exercise does not have to be in a gym and does not have to involve spending hours and hours a day training. It can be incorporated into everyone's lifestyle. It is well known that everyone should engage in physical activity regularly in order to keep themselves fit and healthy.

There are two main components to a weight-loss programme:

- Cardiovascular – this is exercise that gets the heart and lungs working. Cycling, walking, running, swimming etc. will help you burn fat while improving the function of your heart and lungs.
- Resistance training – any training that involves using a load (a weight) to challenge the body. The more traditional forms of weight-bearing exercise use the weight of your body against gravity for resistance, e.g. press-ups, pull-ups and squats. All of these exercises are hugely versatile and great for helping lose weight, and the beauty is that you can do them at the gym or at home.

Classes

Group exercise classes can be highly motivating because of both the instructor and the other class participants, and of course they can be done anywhere, from a gym or studio to outdoors in a park or any open area.

Classes that are suitable for weight loss vary from aerobics or cycling to toning classes using weights. Circuit training is another great way to help you burn fat and tone specific areas.

Sports

Playing sport and games is one way of keeping exercise fun. Not only will it keep you active but there is also the social aspect of training and playing in a team that encourages you to stick at it.

Active Living

As well as 'training' you can exercise in other ways that can be built into your life. Walking is one of the easiest exercises to build into everyday life. Walk to work instead of driving or getting public transport. Use your lunch break as an opportunity to get some exercise. Take the stairs not the lift, walk to the local shops and cycle instead of using the car. You may not think of these things as exercise but they all increase your heart rate, get the blood pumping and burn calories.

Now that you've been convinced of how important physical activity is to your health and well-being, the next step is incorporating it into your life. This is really just a matter of following some simple steps – in fact, you are probably already more physically active than you might think!

Increase Your Activity Levels

The simple fact is that the more calories you use and the less you consume the more weight that you will lose. Some people find that it is hard to exercise enough to lose weight, and find it even harder to commit to enough time to exercise. Here are some tips to help you with this.

- Having clear goals is very important as you will struggle to get anywhere if you do not have an understanding of where you want to go.
- Have smaller goals along the way to help you to reach your main goal. Bite-size goals do not have to be just smaller versions of the bigger one, though. Keep things interesting and mix up your goals – e.g. running 10 minutes longer or cycling a distance in under a certain time. Although these may not be the same as your weight-loss goal, they will help you eventually to achieve it.
- Make sure that the goal you set is achievable and realistic for you. If it is not, you will be left feeling you have failed. To help you in this, write it down!

- Get support from family and friends to help you stay motivated.
- Find the exercise that works for you, experimenting with different types of exercise to find the one that you enjoy the most.

So, work out what you want to achieve, and how you can measure your success along the way.

It is easy to think, I will exercise tomorrow, I am tired today, or I will start again next week. Do it now! Making sure that exercise is in your diary several times a week is very important. Make sure that exercise is not an afterthought but is booked as an important part of your day.

Which Exercise Is Best For Me?

There are many theories behind the best exercise for losing weight, but there are some fundamentals to any routine. Firstly, the exercise must always be a challenge. Secondly, a routine should include both resistance or weight-bearing and cardiovascular exercises.

- Resistance training is a very important part of any exercise routine and, unfortunately, sometimes the most overlooked. One of the main points is that resistance training will help your body gain lean muscle, which will not only look great but also increase the body's energy intake or basal metabolic rate, making it easier for you to control your weight.
- Cardiovascular training has many benefits when it comes to the working efficiency of the heart and lungs. It also has many other benefits, including helping you utilize calories and so lose weight and control it.

Remember, little and often is the best way forward. Improved fitness will allow you to engage in prolonged levels of activity even outside of your exercise programme and with less effort, thus helping you to enjoy an active lifestyle and do more things than you where able to do before.

Cardio and resistance training do not have to be considered separate workouts. A brisk walk after work followed by 10–15 minutes of weight exercises will ensure you optimize weight loss.

Different types of exercise will also burn different amounts of calories. This will be hugely influenced by the intensity of the activity and the time spent doing it. Different people will burn off different amounts of calories depending on their metabolic rate, but below is a table showing an estimate of the calories burned doing some of these activities over an hour.

Exercise	Approximate Number of Calories Burned per Hour
Aerobics, general	422
Aerobics, high impact	493
Badminton	417
Cycling, moderate intensity	563
Cycling, outside moderate	493
Boxing, punching bag	422
Dancing, aerobic, ballet or modern	422
Pushing or pulling buggy with child	176
Rowing, stationary, moderate effort	598
Running, 6mph (10 min mile)	704
Running, 7.5mph (8 min mile)	880
Swimming, backstroke	563
Swimming, breaststroke	604
Tennis	493
Walking, 3mph, mod. pace, walking dog	246
Walking, 3.5mph, uphill	422
Weight-lifting, vigorous effort	422

How to Get the Most Out of Cardio and Resistance Exercise?

You should be looking to incorporate activity into your daily life so that it becomes a habit. Here are some guidelines to help you get started:

- Ensure you are exercising at the right intensity. The easiest and one of the quickest ways to do this is to work out your target heart rate for weight loss. The equation is 220 minus your age. Example: for a 35 year old, 220 – 35 = 185. This tells you the maximum times your heart should beat in a minute. Between 65 and 80 per cent of this is your *target heart-rate zone.*

- You should aim to exercise at least three times a week; however, moderate activity on all days of the week will immensely help you to lose weight and stay active.
- Each training session should last between 20 and 60 minutes to gain significant increases in aerobic fitness and burn a sufficient amount of calories.
- Make sure you include a gradual warm-up before hitting your target heart-rate zone. Steadily build your heart rate for about 5 minutes to prepare your body for exercise.
- For resistance training, ensure you are doing large movements (squats, press-ups, lunges etc.) as these will optimize calorie expenditure.
- When choosing the amount of load or weight to use, be realistic. Your aim should be that the weight is a challenge, but not so heavy for you that your technique is compromised.

This grid shows you an example of the reps (repetitions), sets and recovery you should be aiming for in a typical weight-loss programme.

¾ Press up	2 set
Chest & Shoulders	12–15 reps
	45–30 secs rest

- It is important that a full and correct range of movement is used for all weight-bearing exercises. You cannot get the full benefit of any exercise without working the body through its full range. Correct technique is also very important to avoid injury.

Your Weight-loss Programme

This weight-loss programme will not only help you lose weight but also focus on toning and strengthening specific muscle groups.

The programme involves both cardiovascular and resistance training to maximize weight-loss results.

Remember: it is important to warm up and cool down effectively to avoid injury.

Use this scale to determine the effort level for your work:

1	2	3	4	5
Very light	Light	Moderate	Somewhat heavy	
6	**7**	**8**	**9**	**10**
	Very heavy			Very, very heavy

The RPE scale is used to measure the intensity of your exercise. The numbers above relate to phrases used to rate how easy or difficult you find an activity. For example, 1 (very light) would be how you feel when you are getting up from a chair; 10 (very, very heavy) is how you feel after a very difficult activity.

Terms Used

Rep – This is one complete movement of an exercise. For example if you are completing a squat, it is the going down then coming back up that makes 1 repetition.

Set – A group of repetitions performed together.

Rest – The time in between sets to allow the muscles to recover.

Cardio-vascular		Weeks 1–4	Weeks 5–8	Weeks 9–12
Warm up + Cardio (CV)	Brisk Walk or jog outside or walk on the spot for 3 mins, 2-min jog on the spot and repeat as necessary	5–15 mins RPE 1–6	10–20 mins RPE 1–7	15–25 mins RPE 1–8

Exercise	Teaching Points	Weeks 1–4	Weeks 5–8	Weeks 9–12
Floor Bridge Back of thighs	1. Lie on the floor with knees bent 2. Roll pelvis to flatten back to the floor 3. Drive up through hips as you inhale 4. Hold for a second then lower as you exhale	1 set 12 reps 1 min rest	1–2 sets 12 reps 45 sec rest	2 sets 15 reps 30 sec rest

Exercise	Teaching Points	Weeks 1–4	Weeks 5–8	Weeks 9–12
¾ Press-up Chest & shoulders	1. Adopt a press-up position with your knees on a mat for comfort 2. Keeping a straight line from knee to head gently lower yourself as you inhale 3. Squeeze shoulder blades together at the bottom and press up from the floor as you exhale	1 set 12 reps 1 min rest	1–2 sets 12 reps 45 sec rest	2 sets 15 reps 30 sec rest
Lunge Thighs	1. Stand in a split stance greater and wider than a normal stride 2. Keeping upright, gently lower your body by bending your knees as you inhale, making sure to keep your front heel on the floor 3. Control the bottom position and drive up through the hips as you exhale to return to the start	1 set 12 reps Alternate legs	1–2 sets 12 reps Alternate legs	2 sets 15 reps Alternate legs
Step-ups Pulse raiser	1. Step up and down while keeping the body upright 2. Make sure that the whole foot is placed on the step 3. Remember to either alternate leading foot or change lead foot half way	3 mins RPE 5–6	4 mins RPE 6–7	5 mins RPE 7–8

Exercise	Teaching Points	Weeks 1–4	Weeks 5–8	Weeks 9–12
Chair/ bench squats Front & back of thighs	1. Stand over a chair front with feet shoulder-width apart 2. Keeping the heels on the floor, initiate the movement from the knees, lower the body down towards the chair as you inhale 3. Once you feel the thighs are parallel to the floor, pause briefly 4. Drive up through the feet as you exhale	1 set 12 reps 1 min rest	1–2 sets 12 reps 45 sec rest	2 sets 15 reps 30 sec rest
Ball squats Thighs	1. Stand against a wall with a ball placed in the small of your back and your feet placed just wider than hip width 2. Keeping the body upright, gently lower yourself so that your thighs are parallel to the floor, by rolling down the ball ensuring that the ball supports the lower back throughout 3. Hold briefly, then drive up through the hips as you exhale to the start position	1 set 12 reps 1 min rest	1–2 sets 12 reps 45 sec rest	2 sets 15 reps 30 sec rest
Shoulder press Shoulders	1. Stand in a split stance with your knees bent and two dumb-bells (or cans of beans) at shoulder height 2. Push the dumb-bells overhead in an arc as you inhale while keeping the core strong 3. Hold briefly then lower to the start position as you exhale	1 set 12 reps 1 min rest	1–2 sets 12 reps 45 sec rest	2 sets 15 reps 30 sec rest

Exercise	Teaching Points	Weeks 1–4	Weeks 5–8	Weeks 9–12
Leg reach Back of thighs	1. Stand on 1 leg facing a wall 2. Keeping the chest lifted and tipping from the hips, lean forward to touch the wall as you inhale 3. Hold briefly then return to the start 4. Once this becomes easy, move a couple of inches back to increase the distance	1 set 12 reps Alternate legs	1–2 sets 12 reps Alternate legs	2 sets 15 reps Alternate legs

CV		Weeks 1–4	Weeks 5–8	Weeks 9–12
Cardio (CV) + cool down	Brisk walk outside or walk on the spot to cool down	5–10 mins RPE 6–2	5–10 mins RPE 7–2	5–10 mins RPE 8–2

Hamstring stretch	1. Lie on your back with a towel around one ankle 2. Keeping the back flat on the floor, raise that leg and pull it towards your shoulders so you feel light tension in the back of the leg 3. Hold until the tension eases 4. Repeat with the other leg

Hip flexor stretch	1. Kneel on the floor with one foot in front and other on a mat 2. Place your weight on the lead leg and ease your body forward until you feel gentle tension in the front of the hip of the leg on the floor 3. Hold until the tension eases 4. Swap leg positions and repeat

So now you know what you should be doing, it is just a matter of factoring exercise into your daily life along with your healthy eating plan. Remember we all have time to fit exercise into our lives, it is just a question of prioritizing it so that we actually do it!

Chapter 8

Keep Going!

This chapter is written to encourage you on your journey through weight loss and beyond. It provides guidance on how to cope when you want to give up or hit a weight-loss plateau, and looks to the longer term, suggesting how to maintain your weight loss using successful strategies.

The Power of Your Mind

So much of dieting is related to how you feel. How you feel about yourself, about food and activity, as well as about your ability to succeed. So don't underestimate the power of your mind to boost your efforts – or sabotage them. Giving up will further undermine your self-esteem, at whatever stage of your weight-loss programme, so look for encouragement from as many sources as you can.

If you are feeling tempted to throw in the towel, have a look at the list that follows and find one or more reasons to encourage yourself to go on:

- Find the diet goal you wrote down when you started the diet and remind yourself why you want to lose weight.
- Imagine how good you are going to feel when you are the weight you dream of being.
- If you are part of a support group, ring or mail a friend and chat through your struggles.

- Find a piece of clothing that is now too big and gloat in the fact that it no longer fits.

Also work out why you may be feeling like giving up, and try to address this:

- Did you have a slip-up? Remember that one day's fall from grace is not the end – just get back on track and put it down to experience.
- Are you tired of trying? Don't let the 'apathy voice' in your head get the better of you.
- Does the task ahead seem insurmountable – have you set yourself a realistic goal? Do you need to think about a different or interim goal?
- Are you being kind enough to yourself? Have you rewarded yourself for your progress so far? If not, then do so – buy yourself a magazine, book or some music, or treat yourself to a little pampering.
- You just fancy a pepperoni pizza or fish and chips? Cravings are normal, but try not to get fixated on food. Do something to take your mind off food, and remember the physical and emotional consequences of giving in.
- Have you reached a weight-loss plateau and are discouraged by the lack of progress? Read on!

Reached a Plateau?

If you have been doing really well up till now and your weight loss has ground to a halt, rest assured that this is not unusual when on a diet. It can be very frustrating to find that the weight is not coming off as fast as it was when you have been exercising diligently and sticking to your eating plan.

Why Does It Happen?

While you are dieting you will be decreasing your calories from food, and you should also be burning more calories by increasing your activity levels. (If you are not exercising, herein may lie the problem.) After a while, however, your body gets used to this new regime and your metabolism adjusts. This helps your body protect the fat reserves it has to ward off possible starvation, which of course runs counter to what you want. This means that it is harder to shed weight because your metabolism has settled at a new rate and you reach a plateau in your efforts to lose weight. In order to continue with your weight loss, you'll need to make a few changes to fire up your metabolism a little.

First, check that you are doing all the recommended things:

- Are you still following a diet plan, and writing down what you eat every day?
- Are you sticking to the recommended amount of calories and fat every day?
- Are you still weighing out foods and measuring drinks?
- Are you as active as you were when you first started the diet?

You may find that as you have got used to being on the diet you may have become a bit complacent, so check these things first. If after a week you still haven't shifted any more weight, then it is time for more of a change.

The best way to overcome the plateau is to increase the level and intensity of your physical activity. Change your exercise regime to use some different muscles. Make sure you are doing an activity that is going to strengthen your long muscles (those in your thighs and buttocks). The more lean muscle you have, the more calories they require. If you go to a gym ask the instructors for some help in choosing some new routines.

You could also try to drop the calorie content of your diet a little. For example if you are on the 1600 diet, drop to the 1400 diet for one or two weeks and see if this helps. A drop of even 100 calories may be all that is needed.

Maintaining Your Weight Loss

If you have now reached your target weight, congratulations!

As you know, successful weight loss means keeping the weight off too, so the information that follows should help you maintain your success.

First of all you need to stabilize at your new weight, so you know how many calories your body needs to remain at this weight. This is best done over a period of weeks so you can monitor your weight each week. If you have lost weight on the 1400-calorie plan, then try a week using 1600 calories, weighing yourself at the beginning and end of the week on the same scales. You may find you still lose some weight during the week. If this is the case move up to the 1800-calorie diet for a week or two. If, however, on the 1600-calorie diet your weight remains stable after a week, continue for another week and weigh yourself again. A few weeks with a stable weight at one level will indicate that this is your ideal calorie intake.

Of course it is not just about calories. You know that the healthy diet you were eating was fat controlled, too, so continue to limit the fat in your diet. Read the chapter again on how to eat a healthy diet (pages 17–29) for a quick reminder.

Importantly, you should also continue with your exercise programme – as this, like eating healthily, is a lifelong commitment for weight maintenance. And don't forget to put into practice all the diet and cooking knowledge you have learnt!

Research indicates that dieters who are successful and who keep the weight off employ a range of strategies. None of these will surprise you, as they are sensible, healthy lifestyle changes. The vital fact that makes for their long-term success is commitment and adherence to the changes.

Successful long-term weight maintenance is achieved by:

- continuing to exercise every day
- continuing to eat a lower-fat, restricted-calorie diet
- eating breakfast every day
- having consistent eating patterns, whether weekends or weekdays
- monitoring weight on a regular basis and not allowing modest weight gains to increase.

All of these strategies have been encouraged on the diet, so you should find that once your weight has stabilized you can continue with the great changes you have already chosen. Good luck!

Chapter 9

Portion Guide and Calorie-counter

The tables that follow are have been compiled so that you can put together some meals or snacks yourself by choosing from the many foods shown here. Obviously there are many thousands of foods that could have been included, but the ones here have been selected to give you an average indication of fat and calorie content on a per portion basis. It is a good idea to get used to reading food labels, and there are gaps left in each section so you can add your own favourites.

Portion sizes vary enormously, and average portion sizes and weights are indicated here with a household measure where appropriate. As you get used to weighing and measuring foods for the recipes you will start to become familiar with what a suitable portion looks like for your diet.

The tables also provide limited information on glycaemic index. This is restricted to foods that have been laboratory tested for their GI, so there are several gaps in the data. Foods are shown to have a GI that is either high (least favourable), medium (less favourable) or low (favourable). It is important to remember that foods are not usually eaten in isolation, and the GI can alter when a recipe is put together using a combination of different foods.

Breakfast cereals

Type	size	Portion Wgt g	Fat g	Cal	GI
Cheerios	Ave bowl	40	1.5	147	High
Coco Pops	Ave bowl	30	0.4	115	High
Cornflakes	Ave bowl	30	0.1	106	High
Crunchy Nut Cornflakes	Ave bowl	30	1	121	High
Frosted cornflakes	Ave bowl	30	0.1	113	Low
Muesli, Swiss style	Ave bowl	50	2.9	181	Low
Muesli, with extra fruit	Ave bowl	50	3.1	186	Low
Oatmeal, quick cook, raw	3 tbsp	45	3.9	168	Low
Porridge, made with milk and water	Ave bowl	160	4.9	132	Med
Rice Krispies	Ave bowl	30	0.2	110	High
Shredded Wheat	Ave bowl	40	1.3	146	High
Shreddies	Ave bowl	45	0.6	148	High
Weetabix	Ave bowl	40	0.8	136	High

Breads

Type	size	Portion Wgt g	Fat g	Cal	GI
Wholemeal, medium loaf	1 slice	36	0.9	78	Med
Brown bread, medium loaf	1 slice	36	0.7	78	Med
White bread, medium loaf	1 slice	36	0.6	84	Med
Granary bread, medium loaf	1 slice	36	0.9	84	Med
Multigrain bread, medium loaf	1 slice	51	2.8	115	Med
French bread	5cm slice	40	1	108	Med
White pitta bread	1	75	0.7	153	Med
Wholemeal pitta bread	1	60	1.8	135	
Rye bread	1 slice	25	0.4	54	Low
Bagel	1	80	1.4	218	High
Sesame bagel	1	85	2.5	220	
Cinnamon and raisin bagel	1	85	1.5	221	

Type	Portion size	Wgt g	Fat g	Cal	GI
Currant bread	1 slice	36	2.7	104	Low
Hot cross bun, fruity	1	70	1.1	178	
Hot cross bun, wholemeal	1	70	1.6	171	
Teacake	1	70	2.9	207	
Malt bread	2 slices	35	0.8	93	Low
Rye crispbread	2 crispbreads	20	0.4	72	Med
Wholegrain crackers	1	10	1.2	41	
Tortilla wrap	1	64	2.4	160	
Tortilla wrap, seeded	1	56	3.6	174	

Juices

Type	Portion size	Wgt g	Fat g	Cal	GI
Apple juice unsweetened	200ml glass	200	0.2	76	Low
Carrot juice	200ml glass	200	0.2	48	Low
Cranberry juice, sweetened	200ml glass	200	0	122	Med
Grape juice, unsweetened	200ml glass	200	0.2	92	Med
Grapefruit juice, unsweetened	200ml glass	200	0.2	66	Med
Orange juice, unsweetened	200ml glass	200	0.2	72	Low
Pineapple juice, unsweetened	200ml glass	200	0.2	82	Low
Pomegranate juice, fresh	200ml glass	200	0	88	Med
Tomato juice	200ml glass	200	0	28	Low

Fruits

Type	size	Portion Wgt g	Fat g	Cal	GI
Apple, average eating	medium	100	0.1	47	Low
Apple, average eating	large	150	0.2	70	Low
Apricot, fresh	1	65	0.1	31	Med
Apricots, dried and ready-to-eat	large	40	0.2	63	Low
Avocado	half	75	14.6	142	
Banana	medium	100	0.3	95	Low
Banana	large	150	0.4	143	Low
Dates, fresh	1	25	0	31	High
Grapefruit, raw	half	80	0	24	Low
Grapes	average	100	0.1	60	Low
Kiwi fruit	medium	30	0.3	29	Low
Mango, cubes		100	0.2	58	
Nectarine, with stone	medium	160	0.1	53	
Oranges	medium	160	0.1	59	Low
Peach					
Pear, average	medium	160	0.1	64	Low
Pear, Comice	large	150	0	49	
Pineapple, raw	1 slice	80	0.1	32	Med
Plums, most	medium	55	0	19	Low
Raspberries		100	0.2	25	
Satsuma/clementine	medium	70	0	25	Low
Strawberries		100	0.1	27	Low
Sultanas/raisins/currants	1 tbsp	30	0.1	82	Med

Vegetables

Type	Portion size	Wgt g	Fat g	Cal	GI
Asparagus	5 spears	125	0.7	31	
Beansprouts, raw	1 tbsp	20	0.1	6	Low
Broccoli, boiled	Ave serving	85	0.6	20	
Cabbage, boiled	Ave serving	95	0.3	15	
Carrot, raw	medium	90	0.4	24	
Carrot, boiled	medium	80	0.3	17	Low
Cauliflower, boiled	Ave serving	90	0.8	25	
Celery	1 stick	50	0.1	3	
Cherry tomato	1	15	0.0	2	
Cucumber	quarter	100	0.1	10	
Leek, raw, trimmed	medium	140	0.7	30	
Lettuce, e.g. little gem	half	80	0.4	12	
Mangetout	Ave serving	80	0.0	13	
Mushroom, raw	medium	10	0	1	
Parsnip, boiled	Ave serving	65	0.7	42	High
Pea, frozen	Ave serving	80	0.7	52	
Pepper	half	80	0.3	25	
Swede, boiled	Ave serving	65	0.0	6	High
Sweetcorn, boiled	Ave serving	85	1.9	94	
Spring onion	1	10	0	2	
Tomato, raw	Ave serving	85	0.2	14	
Watercress	¼ bunch	20	0.2	4	

Legumes

Type	Portion size	Wgt g	Fat g	Cal	GI
Baked beans, reheated	3–4 tbsp	135	0.8	113	Med
Broad beans, frozen	2 tbsp	120	0.7	97	High
Red kidney beans	2 tbsp	70	0.4	70	Low

Type	Portion size	Wgt g	Fat g	Cal	GI
Chickpeas, canned	2 tbsp	70	2.0	80	Low
Red lentils, dried, boiled	2 tbsp	80	0.2	80	Low

Starchy Food

Type	Portion size	Wgt g	Fat g	Cal	GI
French fries (McDonald's)	small	n/s	11	230	High
French fries (McDonald's)	medium	n/s	16	330	
French fries (McDonald's)	large	n/s	23	460	
Fries, KFC	regular	n/s	13.2	257	
Fries, KFC	large	n/s	19.4	377	
Oven chips (McCain)	average	200	4.6	272	
New potatoes, boiled	3–4	175	0.5	131	Low
Sweet potato, boiled	small	130	0.3	109	61
Roast potato	3 small	150	6.7	223	High
Baked potato, flesh and skin	small	100	0.2	136	
Baked potato, flesh and skin	medium	180	0.3	244	
Mashed potato, mashed with polyunsaturated spread	3 tbsp	135	5.8	140	
Brown rice, boiled	3 heaped tbsp	120	1.3	169	Low
White rice, easy cook, boiled	3 heaped tbsp	120	1.5	165	Med
White rice, sticky or glutinous, boiled	3 heaped tbsp	120	2.1	171	High
Basmati rice, cooked	3 heaped tbsp	120	0.2	162	Med
Basmati rice, dry	4 level tbsp	50	0.2	180	
Egg noodles, ready soaked	1 pack	150	0.9	244	
Egg noodles, dry, medium	1 nest	65	1.3	224	Low
Couscous, dry weight	4 level tbsp	50	0.1	174	Med
Lasagne, dry sheet	3 sheets	60	1.0	220	

n/s = Not specified

Type	Portion size	Wgt g	Fat g	Cal	GI
Spaghetti or coloured pasta shapes, dry	small	75	1.2	265	Low
Spaghetti or coloured pasta shapes, dry	average	90	1.4	318	
Pasta shapes, cooked	small	150	0.6	219	
Pasta shapes, cooked	average	230	0.9	335	
Egg pasta, dry	average	90	3.2	341	

Dairy food and drink

Type	Portion size	Wgt g/ml	Fat g	Cal	GI
Full fat yogurt, fruit	1 pot	150g	4.5	163	Low
Low-fat (<3% fat) plain yogurt	1 pot	150g	1.5	84	Low
Low-fat (<3% fat) fruit yogurt	1 pot	150g	1.3	135	Low
Greek yogurt (10% fat)	1 pot	150g	15	195	Low
Greek yogurt, fat-free	1 pot	150g	0.1	78	
Soya yogurt, e.g. Alpro plain	1 pot	125g	3.3	67	Low
Virtually fat-free fruit yogurt	1 pot	150g	0.3	70	Low
Skimmed milk	1 glass	250ml	0.7	85	Low
1% fat milk	1 glass	250ml	2.5	97	
Semi-skimmed milk	1 glass	250ml	4.3	115	Low
Whole milk	1 glass	250ml	10	167	
Buttermilk	½ carton	142g	0.7	52	Low
Virtually fat-free fruit fromage frais	rounded tbsp	45g	0.0	22	
Cheese, brie	small piece	40g	11.6	137	
Cheese, cheddar	average	45g	15.5	185	
Cheese, cheddar, reduced-fat	average	45g	7.1	122	
Cheese, stilton	small	40g	14	164	
Cottage cheese	1 tbsp	40g	1.7	40	
Cottage cheese, reduced-fat	1 tbsp	40g	0.6	31	
Mozzarella, buffalo	½ round	67g	14.7	174	
Parmesan, grated	1 dsp	10g	2.9	41	

Type	Portion size	Wgt g	Fat g	Cal	GI
Soft cheese, medium fat	average	30	4.3	53	
Soft cheese, extra light	average	30	1.2	32	
Single cream	1 tbsp	15	2.8	28	
Crème fraîche, reduced-fat	1 level tbsp	15	2.8	29	
Crème fraîche, reduced-fat	1 rounded tbsp	40	7.6	78	
Sour cream	1 level tbsp	15	2.9	30	
Half-fat sour cream	1 level tbsp	15	1.3	18	
Probiotic dairy drink	bottle	100	1.6	72	

Butter and spread

Type	Portion size	Wgt g	Fat g	Cal	GI
Butter, average on bread	average	10	8.2	74	
Olive spread (59% fat)	thinly spread	7	4.3	39	
Olive spread (59% fat)	thickly spread	10	6.2	56	
Olive spread (59% fat)	1 tsp	5	3.1	28	
Polyunsaturated spread (20–25% fat)	thinly spread	7	1.4	12	
Polyunsaturated spread (20–25% fat)	thickly spread	10	2.0	18	
Oil, any type	1 tsp	5	2.9	26	
Oil, any type	1 tbsp	15	10.9	98	
Mayonnaise (full fat)	1 level tbsp	15	11.3	103	
	1 rounded tbsp	45	33.9	309	
Mayonnaise (reduced-fat)	1 level tbsp	15	4.2	43	
	1 rounded tbsp	45	12.6	129	
Caesar dressing	1 tbsp	25	15.8	150	
French dressing	1 tbsp	15	10.8	97	

Nuts

Type	Portion size	Wgt g	Fat g	Cal	GI
Walnuts	6 halves	20	13.7	137	
Peanuts, roasted, salted	¼ bag	50	26.5	301	Low
Almonds	6 almonds	13	7.2	79	
Pinenuts	1 tbsp	15	10.9	110	

Jams, etc.

Type	Portion size	Wgt g	Fat g	Cal	GI
Jam	1 rounded tsp	15	0	39	Low
Marmite	scraping	2	0	3	
Chocolate spread	average	20	7.5	113	
Peanut butter, smooth	thinly spread	12	6.2	72	
Honey	average	20	0	57	

Snack Foods

Type	Portion size	Wgt g	Fat g	Cal	GI
Savoury					
Pretzels, e.g. Boots Shapers mini salted pretzels	bag	25	0.5	95	
M&S giant lightly salted pretzels	¼ bag	50	2.1	190	
Walkers, Baked crisps	bag	25	2.0	97	
Go Ahead crisps	bag	25	4.6	99	
Pringles, average		25	8.5	9	135

Type	size	Wgt g	Fat g	Cal	GI
Kettle crisps	small bag	30	7.7	145	
Breadsticks, average	3	21	1.7	82	
Rice cakes, Sainsbury's BGTY	1	7.7	0.2	29	
Sweet					
Alpen fruit and nut bar	1 bar	28	2.8	111	
Frosties cereal bar	1 bar	25	3.0	103	
Nutrigrain Elevenses, raisin	1 bar	45g	4	164	
Traidcraft Geobar, chocolate and raisin	1 bar	34	1.9	138	
M&S Eat Well Date, Raisin and Oat Cinnamon Bars	1 bar	30	2.9	110	
Kit Kat 2-bar biscuit	1	107	5.6	107	
Digestive biscuit	1 biscuit	13	2.6	60	
Hob Nob mini biscuits, chocolate	1 bag	20	4.7	97	
Ginger biscuit	1 average	11	1.7	50	
Rich Tea, McVities	1	8.4g	1.2	36	
Rocky, chocolate, Fox's	1	24.5	6.6	126	
Toffee popcorn, Butterkist	¼ bag	50	5.0	210	
Custard cream	1	12.6	2.6	63	
Chocolate mini rolls, Sainsbury's	1	29	6.3	136	

Protein-rich foods

Type	size	Wgt g	Fat g	Cal	GI
Chicken breast, grilled, no skin	small	130	2.8	192	
Chicken thigh, skinned and boned, raw	large	100	6.7	135	
Chicken drumstick, roasted with skin	average	42	4.2	86	
Beef, lean mince, raw (<10% fat)	average	130	9.6	226	
Beef, extra-lean steak mince (<5% fat, raw)	average	130	5.8	161	
Pork, diced, lean, raw	average	130	5.2	158	
Pork, chops, loin, lean only, grilled	average	170	8.1	384	

Type	Portion size	Wgt g	Fat g	Cal	GI
Lamb, chops, loin, lean only, grilled	average	70	8.6	155	
Diced lean lamb, Sainsbury's BGTY	½ carton	174.5	5.0	191	
Burger, Tesco Finest Aberdeen Angus	½ carton	170	24.7	365	
Burger, Tesco quarter pounders (frozen)	1	113	12.3	195	
Sausages, Walls classic Cumberland, grilled	2	n/s	16.8	249	
Salmon fillet, raw	1 small	130	18.9	279	
Tuna, canned in water, drained	½ 260g can	130	0.6	149	
Tuna, canned in oil, drained	½ 200g can	92	8.2	173	
Cod fillet, raw	1 small fillet	120	0.8	91	
Fish fingers, grilled Birds Eye	3 fish fingers	90	7.0	165	
Haddock, in batter, deep fried	1 small	170	23.8	394	
Prawns, cooked	average	100	1.4	90	
Ham, premium	1 slice	25	1.2	33	
Ham, wafer thin	4 slices	24	0.6	25	
Eggs, medium, boiled	1	55	5.9	80	
Eggs, 1 medium fried in 1 tsp sunflower oil	1	58	9	106	
Eggs, 1 medium scrambled with 2 tbsp skimmed milk with 1 tsp olive spread,	1	85	9.0	87	

Desserts

Type	Portion size	Wgt g	Fat g	Cal	GI
Chocolate mousse, M&S Count On Us	1 pot	70	1.9	80	
Chocolate mousse, Cadbury	1 pot	55g	4.5	110	
Apple pies, Sainsbury's Basics	1	46.5	7.5	180	
Mince pies, deep filled	1	66.5	9.3	247	
Custard, ready-made low-fat (Ambrosia)	1/3 can	140	2.5	130	
Fruit fool, Tesco strawberry	1 carton	114	12.3	185	
Panna cotta, Sainsbury's	1 carton	120	15.7	335	
Tiramisu, Sainsbury's	1 pot	100	9.9	280	

Type	Portion size	Wgt g	Fat g	Cal	GI
Bread and butter pudding, home made	average	170	13.2	272	
Trifle, e.g. Tesco strawberry	1 pot	150	7.7	190	
Apple crumble	average	170	11.7	351	
Ice cream, dairy, vanilla	125ml	125ml	5.8	117	
Cornetto, classic, Walls	1 cone	60g	11	190	
Choc ice, milk chocolate	1	n/s	8.8	135	

n/s = Not specified

Chocolate

Type	Portion size	Wgt g	Fat g	Cal	GI
Milk chocolate		25	7.6	130	
Mini egg, Cadbury	1	3.3	0.7	15	
Treat-size dairy milk, Cadbury	1	14	4.2	74	
Truffle, vanilla, Thorntons	1	13	3.5	64	
Dairy Milk, Cadbury	49g	49g	13.4	250	
Dark, extra fine, M&S	1 square	13g	5.9	7.2	
Ferrero Rocher	1	12.5g	5.1	7.4	

The information has been taken from manufacturers' data, which is available on the internet and from the standard UK food-composition tables (HMSO/OPSI, *McCance and Widdowson's The Composition of Foods*: 6th edn; 5th edn plus supplements).